Therapy To Go

Therapy To Go

Gourmet Fast Food Handouts for Working with Child, Adolescent and Family Clients

Clare Rosoman

Jessica Kingsley Publishers
London and Philadelphia

First published in 2008
by Jessica Kingsley Publishers
116 Pentonville Road
London N1 9JB, UK
and
400 Market Street, Suite 400
Philadelphia, PA 19106, USA

www.jkp.com

Copyright © Clare Rosoman 2008

Library of Congress Cataloging in Publication Data

Rosoman, Clare.
    Therapy to go : gourmet fast food handouts for working with child, adolescent and family clients / Clare Rosoman.
        p. cm.
    ISBN 978-1-84310-643-2 (pb : alk. paper)
    1. Child psychiatry--Problems, exercises, etc. 2. Adolescent psychiatry--Problems, exercises, etc. 3. Family psychotherapy--Problems, exercises, etc. 4. Patient education. I. Title.
    RJ499.32.R67 2008
    618.92'89--dc22

                                        2008014823

British Library Cataloguing in Publication Data
A CIP catalogue record for this book is available from the British Library

ISBN 978 1 84310 643 2

Printed and bound in Great Britain by
Printwise, Haverhill

Menu

APPETISERS 7

How to use this book 7

Why worksheets? 8

Clinical issues 9

About the author 10

Acknowledgements 10

Starters

SECTION 1 – GETTING STARTED 13

1.1 Rapport building 13

1.2 Boundaries and goals for therapy 20

1.3 Unfolding the story 29

SECTION 2 – THERAPY BASICS 37

2.1 Exploring and expressing emotions 37

2.2 Monitoring 46

2.3 Cognitive behavioural therapy (CBT) 52

2.4 Emotional regulation 64

2.5 Goal-setting 70

2.6 Problem-solving 77

Main Course

SECTION 3 – ANXIETY ISSUES   85

    3.1   Psycho-education and increasing awareness   85

    3.2   Anxiety reduction strategies   93

    3.3   Cognitive behavioural strategies for anxiety   101

SECTION 4 – DEPRESSIVE ISSUES   107

    4.1   Psycho-education   107

    4.2   Behavioural strategies for depression   113

    4.3   Cognitive strategies for depression   119

SECTION 5 – ANGER ISSUES   122

    5.1   Psycho-education   122

    5.2   Motivation for managing anger   129

    5.3   Anger management   135

SECTION 6 – COMMUNICATION SKILLS   140

    6.1   Friendships   140

    6.2   Assertiveness   160

    6.3   Safety and empowerment   172

Dessert

SECTION 7 – FAMILY ISSUES   189

    7.1   Family story   189

    7.2   Connectedness   197

    7.3   Parenting   204

    7.4   Problem-solving   219

SECTION 8 – RESILIENCE   227

    8.1   Building self-esteem   227

    8.2   Body image   233

    8.3   Staying on track   243

APPETISERS

How to use this book

This book is designed to be a quick and easy 'fast food' resource for all kinds of therapists working on a professional level with children, adolescents or families. Whether you trained as a counsellor, psychologist, social worker, family therapist, psychiatrist, child worker or psychotherapist there are activities in this book that can help all therapists to work towards their therapeutic goals with their clients. This book provides fast 'take-away' activities that cover a wide variety of presenting problems. Each activity is presented in worksheet format and can be photocopied for therapists' use with their clients.

The worksheets intend to compliment or expand upon the treatment plan that has already been determined by the client and the therapist. This book is not designed to be a treatment manual and the sheets are not designed to be used in any particular sequence. Rather, it aims to be a stimulus for ideas and creativity in therapy. It is intended that the therapist will pick and choose amongst the worksheets, selecting those activities that will help them to best meet the therapeutic goals.

It is assumed that the professionals using this book have a sound grounding in counselling and diagnostic skills. The book aims to offer a wealth of ideas for activities and techniques to use with clients, so reducing the preparation time for sessions. For therapists of all levels of experience, it offers suggestions for different, creative approaches to difficult client issues and can help avoid the need to develop therapy resources, which can be time-consuming.

To receive the most from this resource, it is helpful to peruse the worksheets to become familiar with them, then to select the activity or a range of activities that are likely to suit the client's presenting concerns. This means that the therapist can take a flexible approach to each session by having a variety of exercises available to use, and can therefore allow the client to determine the direction of discussion. This is especially useful for younger children who need a variety of activities to hold their attention and an assortment of formats to convey a point.

At the start of each section there is an explanation of each activity, including a description of how the sheet could be used in therapy and which age group it is recommended for (children or adolescents). For the purposes of these guides, children are defined as 5–12 years of age and adolescents are between 13 and 18 years. However, this serves as a rough guide only and the therapist will know best which activities will be appropriate for each individual client.

Why worksheets?

Worksheets are a valuable therapeutic tool because they are visual, direct and structured. They vary the process of therapy and can provide a framework for the content of a therapy session. This book aims to compile a large amount of commonly needed therapy tools in order to save the therapist time and to provide immediate 'take-away' ideas to be used with their clients.

For the child and adolescent client, worksheets are easy to read and are visually appealing. They are non-threatening because they contain limited amounts of information and they can be worked through to the client's self-determined level of comfort. They provide a sense of safety because the client can see the activity or questions before they commence and can feel in control of how deeply they expose themselves.

Worksheets can guide the content and process of therapy by opening up discussion and exploring deeper issues that the client may feel happier writing down or thinking about first. The sheets in this book aim to provide a variety of ideas to help therapists to guide their client's discovery.

One of the values of worksheets is that they can be taken home by the client. This means that the information contained on the worksheets can be digested over time and taken out of the therapy room to be read and re-read, stuck up on the wall as a visual prompt, or can be shown to friends and family members. This may encourage the generalisation and inter-contextualisation of therapeutic progress.

This is, after all, what therapy is all about: applying the therapeutic strategies to life outside of the therapy room.

Clinical issues

The worksheets and activities in this book aim to assist the therapist in:

- forming rapport with the client and hearing the client's story
- determining treatment goals and the client's motivation to change
- using specific techniques to explore the client's experiences
- educating the client about psychological constructs
- motivating the client
- helping the client to gain insight and to develop as a person
- improving the client's interpersonal relationships, coping ability, and building their resilience.

These worksheets can be used to enhance or guide treatment of a variety of problems, including:

- depression and mood disorders
- anxiety disorders, including generalised anxiety disorder, specific and social phobias, post-traumatic stress disorder, panic disorder, obsessive compulsive disorder, as well as worry and perfectionism
- anger and behavioural issues
- interpersonal issues, including poor communication, bullying, lack of assertiveness, inadequate social skills and low confidence
- eating and body image concerns
- family and parenting difficulties
- low self-esteem, lack of direction and focus in life, lack of goal-achievement.

About the author

Dr Clare Rosoman (née Whiting) is a clinical psychologist currently managing a large not-for-profit psychology clinic in Queensland, Australia. Additionally, she is a consultant at Griffith University as a supervisor of postgraduate clinical psychology students in their work with clients. Clare received her Bachelor of Psychology with Honours from the University of New England and her Doctor of Psychology (Clinical) from Griffith University, Brisbane. Since graduating she has worked in a variety of settings, including psychiatric hospitals, private practice, schools and universities. She is strongly interested in and has been active in the training of therapists such as psychologists and psychiatry registrars. She has had several papers published in the area of children's social functioning and antisocial behaviour.

She recognised a need for a resource for therapists that contained easy-to-use, simple worksheets from the fervour her students displayed in photocopying her folders of collected sheets. As a resource, this book represents years of accumulated therapy tools in one easy location. For training therapists, it provides security in the form of a tool-kit and for more experienced therapists it avoids reinventing the wheel when a resource is needed for a session.

Acknowledgments

These activities and worksheets have been inspired by many theories and schools of thought in psychology, counselling and psychiatry. Many of the exercises draw from the principles of cognitive behavioural therapy (CBT), narrative therapy and solution-focused therapy as well as the accumulated knowledge and wisdom of many practitioners. The author wishes to acknowledge the work of these amazing theorists and practitioners and to emphasise that these worksheets represent a pooling of a vast wealth of shared knowledge and understanding in the practice of psychotherapy.

STARTERS

1 GETTING STARTED

1.1 Rapport building

Building rapport with child and adolescent clients is vital to the success of the therapeutic relationship. If the client trusts their therapist and feels that they can trust them with their feelings, then therapy is given the utmost chance of being significant and productive. The worksheets in this section all aim to put the client at ease, to build trust in the therapeutic relationship, and to allow the therapist to show an unconditional positive regard for the child or adolescent client.

Introducing ME!

Suitable for: any age

This sheet is designed to encourage non-threatening discussion about the client. It has a purely positive focus to create a feeling of safety and acceptance for the client and plenty of opportunities for the therapist to provide warmth and validation. It can be helpful for the therapist to complete one of these sheets at the same time as the client so that each can get to know the other. Of course, the therapist would limit how much they choose to disclose in this exercise and would make sure that the main focus is on the client. However, by being willing to complete the same activity that the therapist asks the client to complete, the therapist sets a safe, fair and non-threatening tone for therapy and models a willingness to contribute to the therapeutic relationship.

Amazing Me

Suitable for: any age

In this activity, children and adolescents are asked to draw themselves and to describe some of the parts of their life, such as their hobbies, interests, friends, family, etc. This might be a light and non-threatening way to find out about their activities and might lead to topics of conversation they feel comfortable with, thus building rapport before beginning to talk about the 'problem'. Special hobbies or interests might be important for the therapist to note early on in therapy because they might serve protective functions or be useful in treatment planning. For example, a child who loves to listen to music could use this as a relaxation or de-escalation strategy later in therapy.

My House

Suitable for: children

In this exercise the client is asked to draw their house for the therapist, describing and drawing all of the people who live there. Some children will prefer to draw the outside of their house and others will draw the floor plan. Whatever the client decides to focus on will give the therapist lots of information about the child's family and their role in the family.

A Bit about Me

Suitable for: adolescents

This sheet is suitable for older children and adolescents because it encourages a deeper level of disclosure and it is a written task. It is valuable because it allows the therapist and the client to explore more deeply, but always at the client's level of comfort.

Introducting ME!

My name is: _____

My birthday sign is: _____

Some of my favourite things are...

- favourite TV program: _____

- favourite food: _____

- favourite pastime: _____

- favourite holiday destination: _____

If I could be an animal I would be _____

because _____

_____

If I had a million dollars I would:

_____

_____

Three things I am good at:

_____

_____

_____

Amazing Me

In the box below draw yourself. In the circles around you, put in your favourite things to do, your favourite people and any other part of your life.

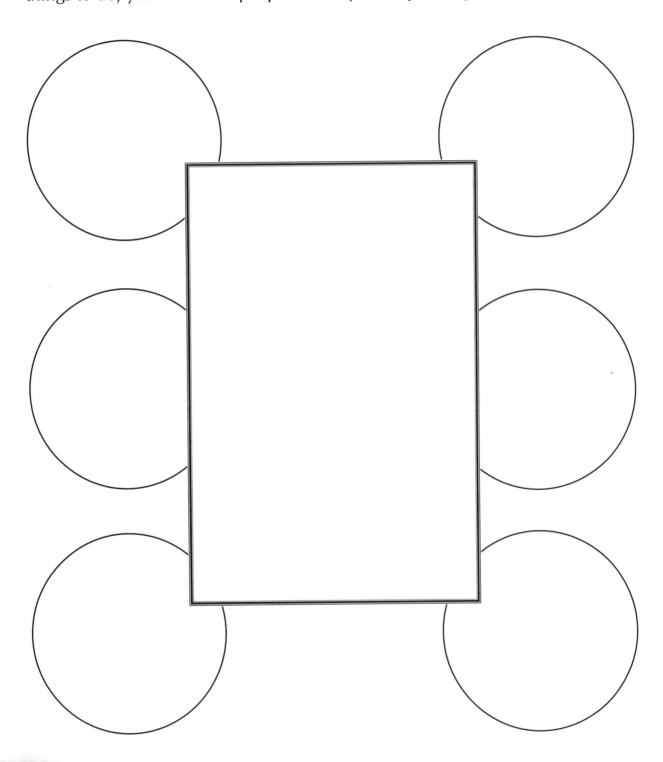

My House

Draw your house below! Include all of the people who live there and the things that you do there.

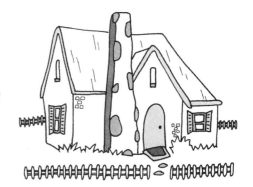

A Bit about Me

My favourite thing is _____

_____

_____

Growing up for me has been _____

_____

_____

What I like about me is _____

_____

_____

Thinking into the future _____

_____

_____

Thinking about the past _____

_____

_____

People around me are _____

_____

_____

I wish _____

_____

_____

The best thing for me _____

_____

_____

One day I would like to _____

_____

_____

I wish people would _____

_____

_____

1.2 Boundaries and goals for therapy

At the beginning of therapy it is important for the child and adolescent client to have a clear idea of the boundaries around the therapeutic relationship. Young people need to be very clear about what the therapist can and cannot keep confidential, what they will have to do in therapy, and how much control they will have over the therapeutic relationship. This will help them to feel safe, respected and open to change.

Confidentiality Form

Suitable for: any age

This form outlines the nature and limits of confidentiality for the child or adolescent child. This is important for the parents/guardians to be aware of as well, particularly regarding their child's safety. It is vital that both the client and their parents are fully apprised of the limits of confidentiality and that parents know that the therapist will not be automatically telling them all that is disclosed in therapy by their child. This is very important for building trust with adolescent clients, who will need to feel that the therapist is aligned with them rather than their parents. That said, it is reassuring for parents to know that the therapist will be alerting them if there are safety issues and that they will be included in their child's treatment as much as possible.

Boundaries

Suitable for: any age

This is an informative sheet used to describe what boundaries are for adolescents and children. It uses a simple 'wall' analogy that can be extended to all relationships in the client's life, but particularly to explain that the therapeutic relationship is a special relationship with the thickness of the wall being decided entirely by the client and their comfort level. This can help with limit-setting for young clients who might want to find out personal information about the therapist or who might be at risk of becoming overly dependent upon the therapist.

Magic Wand

Suitable for: any age

This is an unstructured approach to therapeutic goal-setting and can give startling insights into the client's life and expectations. It involves asking the client what they would change in their life if they had a magic wand. This can be used with any age-group and to any level of depth, thus it can warrant light, superficial information (non-threatening) or can provide deeper discussion about the client's life situation.

Three Wishes

Suitable for: any age

This is a sheet that encourages clients to think of three wishes they have. This can be used with a broad (any wishes they have) or narrow focus (wishes for therapy) to gain insight into the client's goals for change in their life.

Narrative Therapy Questions

Suitable for: any age

This is a list of therapeutic questions in the narrative therapy framework that encourages children to see the 'problem' as an entity external to themselves. It aims to gradually build a narrative where the problem is given a name and its characteristics explored so that the child can see it as a 'monster' to be beaten. This is a creative way of looking at a problem and has been found to greatly enhance the motivation of children to 'fight' their particular 'monster'. (For more information see J. Freeman, D. Epston and D. Lobovits (1997) *Playful Approaches to Serious Problems: Narrative Therapy with Children and Their Families.* New York: Norton.)

This list of questions is designed for the therapist to ask the child client rather than the child reading through the list. As the narrative is woven, therapy can then focus on drawing their monster and then on beating it. For adolescents, a less monster-driven form of externalisation could be used by simply calling the problem 'anger' or 'fear', etc. For instance, the therapist could ask, 'How does fear take over your life?' This is a little more age-appropriate for teens and less likely to be seen as 'kids' stuff'.

Children and adolescents work extremely well by externalising the problem and seeing it as an enemy to be fought. This way they can feel less to blame and can use their avid imaginations in beating the problem. This forms a perfect platform for then teaching the child various skills to tackle their problem and stop it from 'winning'. It is important that parents understand the rationale behind the analogy so that they can best support therapy. This approach makes therapy less threatening, more fun and a manageable challenge for the young client. In this way, the therapist becomes the coach who stands with the child and helps to empower them to fight their problem.

Confidentiality Form

Therapy is confidential...

WHAT DOES 'CONFIDENTIAL' MEAN?

Confidential means that all information shared during therapy will be *kept private*. That means that I can't tell anyone about the things you tell me during our sessions without *your permission first*.

BUT...there are some exceptions

I am *obliged by law* to break confidentiality and tell someone *without your permission* if:

- I am concerned that you may be going to harm yourself (deliberately hurt yourself in any way, or attempt suicide)

- I am concerned that someone is hurting/harming you (verbal/emotional abuse; sexual abuse; physical violence)

- I am concerned that you may be going to do something illegal, or harmful to another person

- if I have to give my records to a court of law.

If I have to break confidentiality, *I will always try to tell you first*.

Then, I am required to tell your parents or another adult who is responsible for you.

I would *always prefer us to tell your parents/guardian together*.

Boundaries

Boundaries are like an imaginary fence we all have around ourselves that marks out where our personal space begins and another's ends – like a fence around your house.

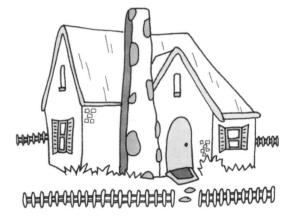

This sort of boundary is a **personal boundary** that controls how close you let others get to you (both physically and emotionally).

The closer you are to a person, the thinner, lower or more see-through your fence is with that person. This means that you let them closer to you **physically** (hugs/touching) and **emotionally** (share more of your feelings and secrets).

For instance, you would have a broader boundary (brick wall) with someone you had just met, and would probably not share as much of yourself as you would with your mother (thin wire fence).

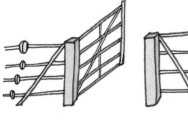
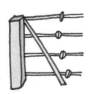

Who in your life do you have a very open boundary with? Who are you closest to of all the people in your life? Who knows the most about you?

_____

_____

_____

Who do you have a medium boundary with? Who knows some things about you but not everything?

_____

_____

_____

Who do you have a big, thick boundary with? Who do you never let in at all?

_____

_____

_____

Magic Wand

If you could wave a magic wand and change your life, what would you change?
Write these things around the wand!

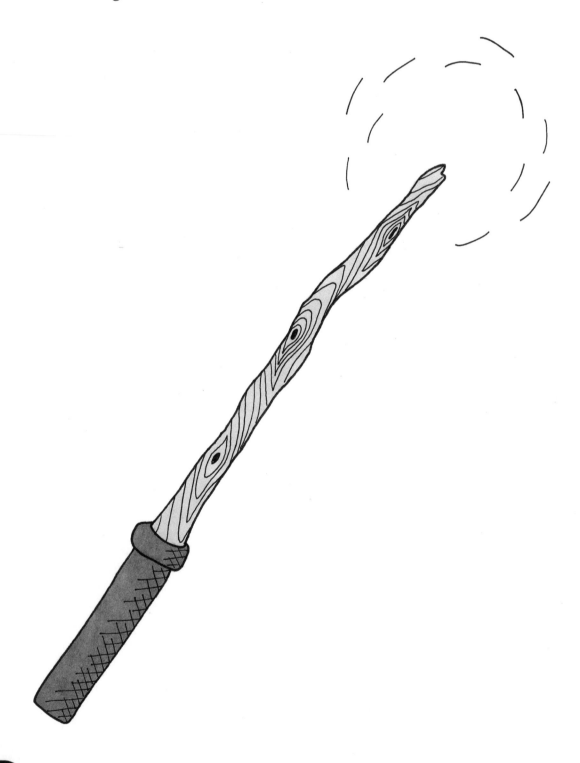

Three Wishes...

My first wish is...

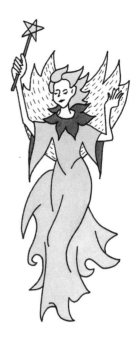

My second wish is...

My third wish is...

Narrative Therapy Questions

What could we call the problem? (e.g. Scaredy Cat, Terrible Temper, Cranky Pants, Sad Sack, Shy Baby, Hot Head, Worry Guts, Cheeky Chicken etc.)

What does he/she like to do to you?

How do you know when he/she is around?

How can you tell when he/she is sneaking up on you?

How does he/she take away your fun?

How does he/she get you into trouble?

How old does he/she make you feel?

What does he/she stop you from doing?

When is he/she most often around?

What things does he/she whisper in your ear?

How do you make her/him go away?

What does he/she make you do?

Do you like having her/him in your life?

What would your life be like without her/him in it?

What could you do if he/she wasn't in your life?

How old would you feel if he/she wasn't around?

Have you ever defeated him/her? How?

What could we do together to help you beat him/her?

Would you like us to try?

1.3 Unfolding the Story

Once the young client and their caregiver understand the process and boundaries of therapy, the initial presenting problem has been discussed, and the client's goals for change have been assessed, it is time to gather information about the client's life to date. This will often involve gaining information from the parents/caregivers as well as the client and may also involve talking to other parties involved in the client's life (such as the school). The forms in this section provide some different options for gaining a thorough understanding of the client's history.

My Storybook

Suitable for: children

This sheet allows the client to tell their story in the manner of a storybook. There is room for illustrations and as much or as little text as needed by the client to tell their own story. It will be necessary to duplicate and perhaps enlarge the page so that the client has plenty of room to record their story on as many pages as needed. Children particularly like to create a story that conceptualises their life and their concerns with themselves as the hero or heroine. This story can then be added to throughout therapy so that it contains strategies and positive outcomes (the inevitable happy ending!). This will then be a useful revision tool.

Personal History – Early Childhood

Suitable for: any age

This is a more structured form that could be used as an intake form for the client's parent/caregiver to complete before their first session, or as a prompt for the therapist while conducting the intake interview with a child or adolescent client and a parent/caregiver. It focuses specifically on early childhood development (up until age 10).

Personal History – Late Childhood/Adolescence

Suitable for: adolescents

This form follows on from the above and focuses on late childhood and adolescence (from age 10–18).

Where I've Come from and Where I'm Going

Suitable for: older children and adolescents

This sheet allows the therapist to formulate the client's presenting problem by examining the factors that set the scene for the presenting problem to surface (predisposing factors), the factors that brought it to a head currently or recently (precipitating factors) and the factors that are maintaining the presenting problem in the client's life (perpetuating factors).

By presenting this to the client and their family this exercise is highly validating and helps all parties to gain increased insight into the client's issues. This then prepares the client and their family for treatment and allows the therapist to present their rationale for treatment (how it will address the maintaining factors and work through predisposing and precipitating factors). It is best if the therapist works through the formulation before presenting it to the client and their family so that it can be done in a clear and positive manner, while still remaining collaborative and open to adjustments.

My Storybook

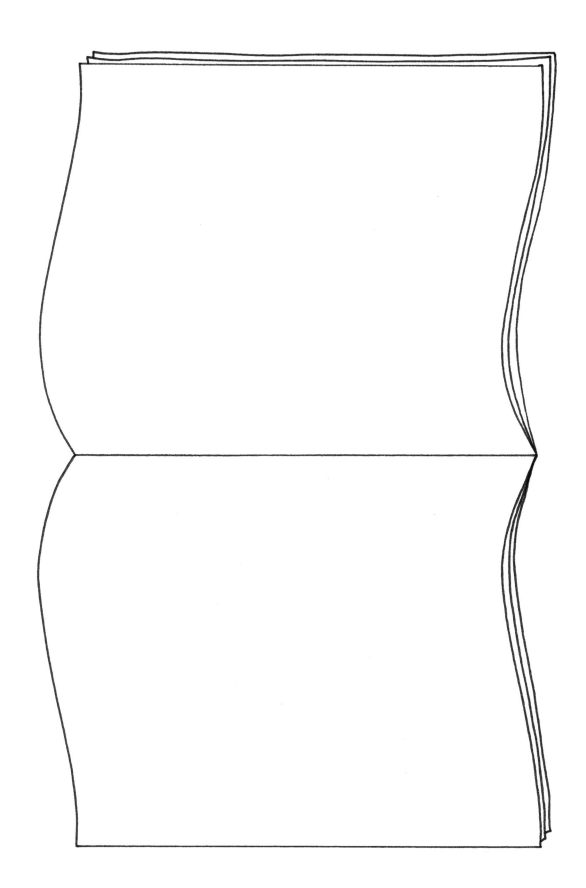

Personal History – Early Childhood

Family details:

Mother: _____   Father: _____

Step-parents/other caregivers: _____

_____

Siblings: _____

_____

Who does your child currently live with?

_____

_____

If your child visits one parent regularly, what are the arrangements for this?

_____

Describe your child's pre-natal and postnatal development – up to six months _(including any complications, temperament, milestones)_:

_____

_____

Describe your child's early childhood – up to three years _(including their interaction in the family, childcare, milestones, any problems)_:

_____

_____

How did your child manage in their preschool/kindergarten years – up to five years *(include socially, separating from you, being in new environments)?*

_____

_____

_____

Describe your child's interaction in the family from age five to the present *(include information on interaction with parents and siblings)*:

_____

_____

_____

Describe your child's experience at school up to age ten *(academically and socially)*:

_____

_____

_____

When did these problems begin and what do you think contributed to them?

_____

_____

_____

Personal History – Late Childhood/Adolescence

Describe your observation of your child's transition from childhood to adolescence:

_____

_____

_____

How have the difficulties developed or changed as they have grown older?

_____

_____

_____

Describe your child's relationship with each parent/caregiver:

_____

_____

_____

Describe your child's experience at school up to the present *(academically and socially)*:

_____

_____

_____

What is your biggest concern for your child?

_____

_____

_____

What would you like for them to gain from coming to therapy?

_____

_____

_____

Have you sought any help for your child before? If so, where, and what was the outcome?

_____

_____

_____

Is your child on any medication *(list names and dosages and period of time pre-scribed)*?

_____

_____

_____

Where I've Come from and Where I'm Going

The main issues that are causing difficulty are:

⬇

The factors that set the scene for the development of these issues are:

⬇

The factors that set it off or brought it to a head are:

⬇

The factors that are maintaining these difficulties are:

⬇

What is our plan to tackle these issues?

SECTION 2 THERAPY BASICS

2.1 Exploring and expressing emotions

This section contains a variety of activities and exercises to encourage children and adolescents to explore emotions and to think about how emotions impact upon their lives. These worksheets will help the therapist to gain some insight into the client's emotional awareness and sensitivity to their own emotions as well as those of others.

Emotions for Kids!

Suitable for: children

This is a basic emotions sheet that lists four major emotions and includes pictures to help children identify them. This sheet asks children to connect the feeling with the accompanying facial expression. It can be used to clarify children's understanding of the names of the emotions and their experience of the different emotions. Sometimes, children may be confused about the subtleties of the different feelings, so this simple exercise allows the therapist to assess their understanding and to discuss the differences between the feelings with them. This can lead to discussion about when they feel each of the listed feelings, why, and what happens in their body and behaviour when they experience each feeling.

Pick a Feeling

Suitable for: children

This sheet encourages children to think about the feelings they experience in different situations. It aims to emphasise the link between situations and feelings, with a view to later discussion about the role of thoughts in emotions. It helps the therapist to gain insight into the child's feelings and their general emotional understanding and cognitive awareness. This sheet can be useful for adolescent clients as well, for the same reasons.

Reading the Signs

Suitable for: children

This exercise is especially aimed at younger children. It contains drawings of people and asks the client to guess what feeling each person is expressing. This creates discussion with children about facial expressions and body language and can highlight whether the child client has difficulty in reading others' moods and expressions. This can give the therapist important information regarding the child's social skills and empathy.

Understanding Emotions

Suitable for: older children and adolescents

This exercise looks in detail at one specific emotion that causes problems for the child or adolescent client. It helps them to examine all of the physical manifestations of that particular emotion, as well as looking at the positives and negatives of that emotion. Finally, this sheet introduces the idea of triggers for that particular emotion in order to increase awareness and to prepare for mood management strategies.

My Feelings

Suitable for: adolescents

This worksheet can be worked through in session or for homework and encourages the client to think about their feelings and the impact of them on their life. It can be used with older children and adolescents as a written exercise and with young children as a dialogue. It is useful because it can provide the therapist with valuable information regarding the most prominent emotions causing problems for the client. This also helps the client to objectively review the emotions that cause them the most difficulty.

Feelings Bubbles

Suitable for: any age

This sheet encourages the client to reflect upon which feelings they experience rarely, sometimes, and often. This is especially useful for children and adolescents in helping them identify which feelings cause the most difficulty for them. This then helps the therapist in developing a treatment plan for the client to tackle the difficult emotions in their life.

Emotions for Kids!

Can you draw a line linking the emotion to the face? When do you feel each of these feelings?

Happy

Sad

Angry

Scared

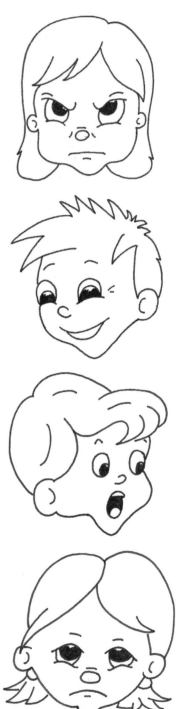

Pick a Feeling

Draw a line from the sentence to the face to show how you would feel if...

Your mum and dad had a fight

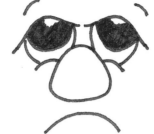

You got in trouble for talking in class

You heard a loud noise in the middle of the night

You weren't allowed to have a friend over to stay

You didn't do your homework and the teacher found out

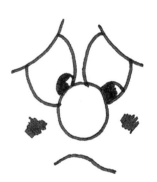

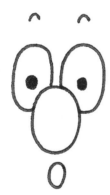

Your best friend stopped talking to you

Some older kids teased you

You had a secret that you couldn't tell anyone about

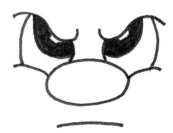

Reading the Signs

Can you guess how these people feel by looking at their facial expressions and how they use their bodies?

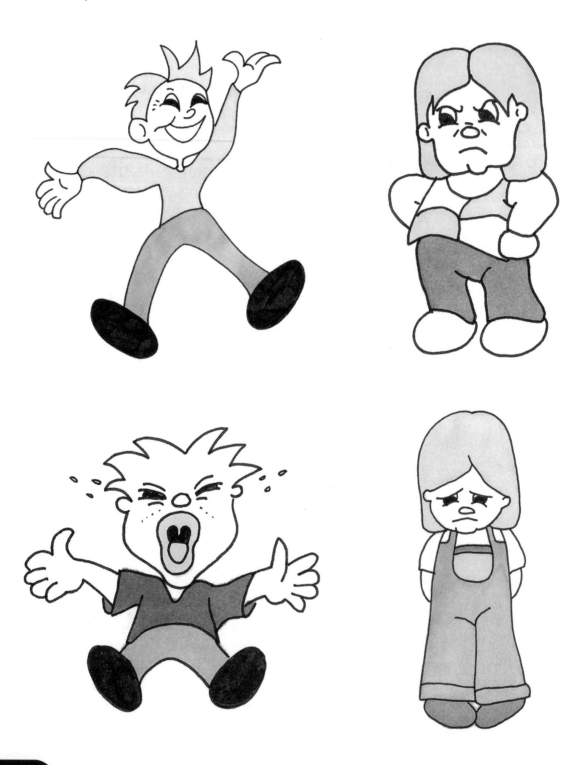

Understanding Emotions

One emotion that causes me problems is: _____

Draw onto the person all the physical feelings related to your emotion, e.g. tight chest, tense muscles, or low energy, etc.

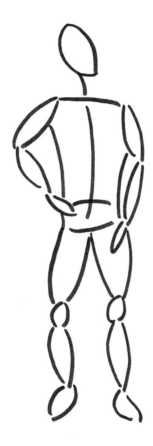

When is this emotion helpful and why?

When is it unhelpful and why?

What things usually happen that cause this emotion?

Copyright © Clare Rosoman 2008

My Feelings

I am happiest when _____

_____

I get scared when _____

_____

I am confused by _____

_____

I feel guilty when _____

_____

I am hurt by _____

_____

I am embarrassed by _____

_____

I am envious of _____

_____

I feel sad when _____

_____

I get angry when _____

_____

Feelings Bubbles

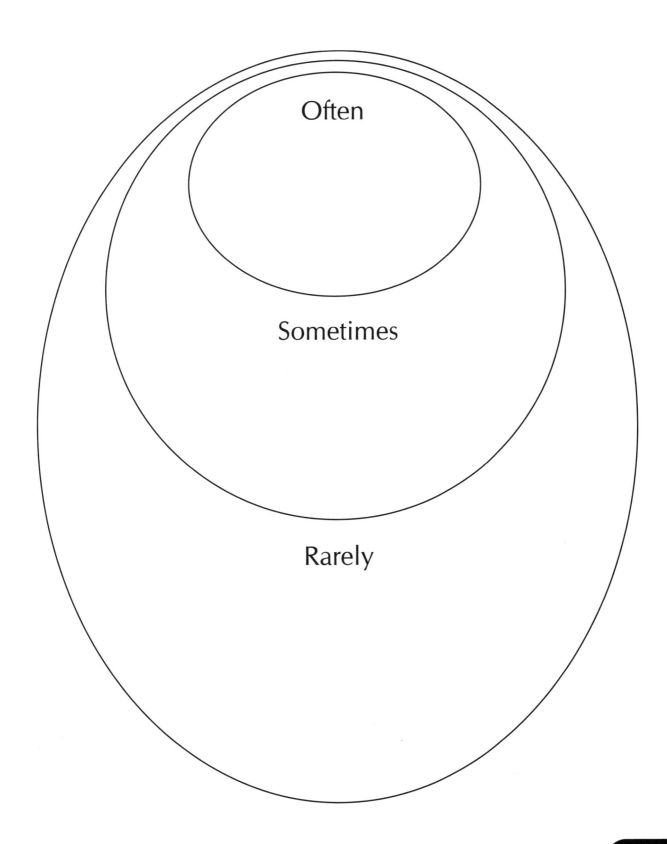

2.2 Monitoring

This section contains some different monitoring sheets to allow the therapist to gain a baseline of the child or adolescent client's presenting issue. In many cases, the parent or caregiver will need to complete these forms to provide reliable data. However, it is also important that children and adolescents become increasingly aware of their feelings and reactions through observation.

Feelings Thermometer

Suitable for: any age

This chart illustrates for the young client a ten-point scale for monitoring emotion. It is a useful tool because it creates a common language between the therapist and the client about the intensity of emotions, as well as providing an objective scale for the client to learn to rate their emotions. Clients of all ages will find this useful.

Activity Recording

Suitable for: any age

This table records the amount of *time* the client engaged in the target behaviour. This is especially useful for the parent to record the length of time the child engaged in the target behaviour, whether that is a positive behaviour that you aim to increase, or a negative behaviour that you aim to decrease through therapy. This monitoring sheet is only useful for target behaviours that are to be *extended* or *shortened* through therapy.

Behavioural Analysis

Suitable for: any age

This monitoring form guides the client through the process of breaking down a problem behaviour into its many components by asking them to observe and record what happened, where and when it happened, what preceded the behaviour and followed the behaviour, and any steps they took to deal with it. This is especially useful for parents/caregivers of children who have targeted a specific problem behaviour in their child that they want to address in therapy. Additionally, this type of form could be useful for adolescents who want to understand more about their target problem behaviour. Monitoring forms such as this one give the therapist valuable information regarding the target behaviour, as well as increasing the client's awareness.

Frequency Observation

Suitable for: any age

This table records the *number of times* a problem behaviour or emotion occurs during a day and compares this over a week. This is valuable for monitoring short-lived problems that occur with a high frequency (e.g. tantrums, swearing, breaking rules, answering back). It allows the therapist and the parent to gain accurate data regarding the frequency of the problem behaviour or emotion and helps all parties to see changes as they are made.

Feelings Thermometer

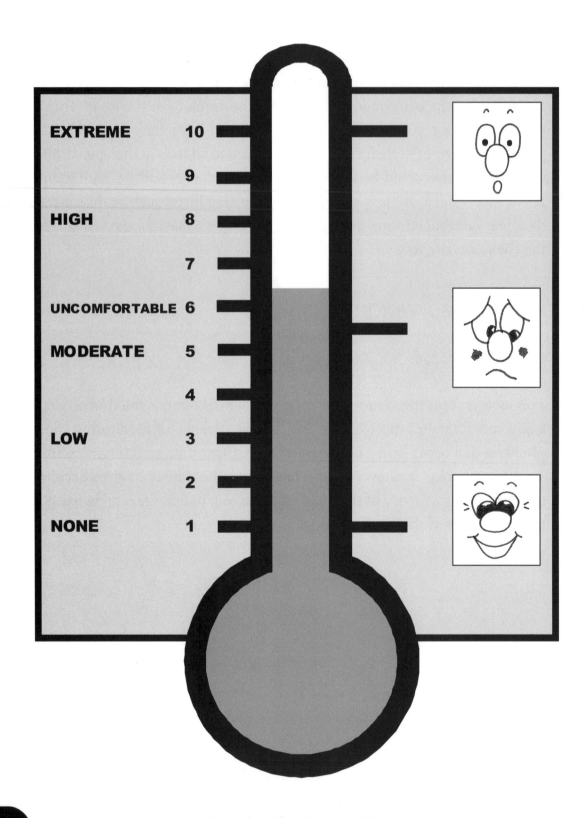

EXTREME	10
	9
HIGH	8
	7
UNCOMFORTABLE	6
MODERATE	5
	4
LOW	3
	2
NONE	1

Activity Recording

Name: _____   **Date:** _____   **Target behaviour:** _____

List below **each time** the target behaviour occurs and for **how long** (in minutes).

Day	mins.	mins.	mins.	mins.	mins.	mins.	mins.	mins.	Daily total
Monday									
Tuesday									
Wednesday									
Thursday									
Friday									
Saturday									
Sunday									

Behavioural Analysis

Name: _____   **Date:** _____   **Target behaviour:** _____

Each time the problem behaviour occurs, write below exactly **what happened**, **where and when** it occurred, what happened immediately **before and after** the behaviour, and what **action** you took to deal with it.

What happened?	Where and when?	What happened before?	What happened after?	What action did you take?

Frequency Observation

Name: _____   **Date:** _____   **Target behaviour:** _____

List below **each time** the target behaviour occurs in a day. Place **one tick** in a box **for each occurrence** on that day.

Day	1	2	3	4	5	6	7	8	9	10	11	12	13	14	15	Daily total
Monday																
Tuesday																
Wednesday																
Thursday																
Friday																
Saturday																
Sunday																

2.3 Cognitive behavioural therapy (CBT)

This section aims to present some of the main ideas and techniques of cognitive behavioural therapy in worksheet format for the child or adolescent client. (See Judith Beck (1995) *Cognitive Therapy: Basics and Beyond*. New York: Guilford Press for more information.) The concepts have been simplified and use age-appropriate examples so that they are easily digestible for young clients.

What is Therapy?

Suitable for: older children and adolescents

This sheet explains what happens when a person begins therapy. In simple language the concepts of CBT are explained, including 'catching and challenging your thoughts' and 'facing your fears in small steps'. When a child or adolescent client understands why the therapist is asking them to complete an activity (particularly if it is uncomfortable), they are far more likely to attempt it and to give it their best effort. Therefore, this sheet forms an introduction to the techniques of CBT and the concepts behind them.

Recording your Thoughts

Suitable for: older children and adolescents

This sheet provides space for the client to practice identifying the events that lead to a negative emotion and/or behaviour. This helps children and adolescents to clearly differentiate between thoughts, emotions and behaviours and to see the powerful effect of thinking on emotions and behaviours. This can be used with adolescents and older children but could be used with younger children if the therapist or parent can help the child.

The Power of Thoughts...

Suitable for: adolescents

This sheet is aimed at adolescent clients and uses an age-appropriate example to illustrate the power of cognitions on mood and behaviour. It aims to pave the way for cognitive restructuring by introducing the role of thinking in emotion.

First Day at School

Suitable for: children

This is similar to the last sheet but uses a younger example to use with younger children to demonstrate the link between thoughts, feelings and behaviour. This can be a written exercise with older children or a talking exercise with younger children. It could be supplemented with snippets from their favourite television program or story book where the therapist asks them what each character is thinking and feeling at certain points and how they could think differently to change how they feel.

Challenging your Thoughts

Suitable for: older children and adolescents

This is a brief list of questions the client can ask themselves to help them to challenge their unhelpful thoughts. It can be helpful to foster an attitude of 'answering back' to negative or unhelpful cognitions to help the young person to feel motivated in fighting their unhelpful thinking. This prepares the client to construct a more realistic and helpful thought to replace the unhelpful one. This can be tailored to the client's level of understanding by using it as an example and then creating the child's own list of ways to answer back to their unhelpful thoughts.

Changing your Thinking

Suitable for: older children and adolescents

This is a more detailed cognitive restructuring sheet that is best suited to adolescents and older children due to its complexity and the written requirement. It coaches the client in identifying unhelpful thoughts, challenging them, and finally generating a more helpful, realistic thought. For younger children, the therapist could help them to make their own list of helpful thoughts that they could tell themselves when they feel upset. These could then be made into a poster or put onto coping cards for the child to carry.

Helpful Thoughts, Unhelpful Thoughts

Suitable for: children

This is a simplified version of the 'Changing your Thinking' sheet, for use with younger children or adolescents who are not as comfortable with the concepts of thought challenging. It simply focuses on identifying unhelpful thoughts and changing them into more helpful, realistic thoughts.

What is Therapy?

- Coming to therapy means that you are very brave and that you want to feel happier with your life and yourself.

- Your therapist is a special person for you to talk to about anything at all that is on your mind.

- Your therapist's job is to listen to you and to give you lots of ideas on how to cope when you feel sad or stressed or upset so that you can feel a bit better.

What do you do in therapy?

- **First**, your therapist will help you to understand what it is that is bothering you and why.

- **Second**, you will learn the difference between thoughts, feelings and behaviours.

- **Third**, you will learn how to change your thoughts to change how you feel.

- **Sometimes**, you will learn how to break your fears down into small steps so that you can overcome them.

- **Other times**, you will learn how to feel better about yourself, how to express how you feel to others, how to manage strong emotions and how to stay calm and happy.

Examples

SUZY

Suzy was very scared all of the time. She was scared about getting sick, about something bad happening to her mother, and about someone breaking into her house at night. She was so worried that she couldn't sleep well, she felt sick in her tummy and she cried a lot.

   When she came to therapy, her therapist helped her to calm her body and to think more helpful thoughts, so that she felt less scared and more positive.

TOM

When Tom came to therapy, his parents were very angry with him because he had been fighting with his sister, had been rude to his parents, and he had been getting into trouble at school. He felt that no-one liked him and that he was always doing the wrong thing.

   Tom's therapist helped him to manage his angry feelings and to be able to express what was bothering him in calm, clear ways. He learned how to feel better about himself and how to do the right things at school. He started to feel much happier.

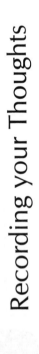

Recording your Thoughts

Event What happened? *e.g. friend broke her promise.*	Thoughts What you actually told yourself. *e.g. 'I can't believe she did that!'*	Emotions Name and rate (0–10). *e.g. angry (8) and anxious (6)*	Behaviour Describe what you did or your body did. *e.g. heart rate increased and I yelled.*

The Power of Thoughts...

What you say to yourself can directly affect your feelings and behaviour in a situation. Your thoughts have huge power over your feelings.

Sally and Kate are going to a party, Sally thinks to herself, 'I am going to have the best night!! I can't wait to arrive, I have my outfit all ready and I know the guy I like is going to be there!!' On the other hand, Kate says to herself, 'I don't really want to go, I know I'm not going to have a very good time. No-one will talk to me, none of the guys ever like me, they always go for Sally. I'm such a loser.'

What emotions would Sally be feeling? Why?

What emotions would Kate be feeling? Why?

How would Sally behave at the party? Would she be likely to have a good time?

How would Kate behave at the party? Would she be likely to have a good time?

What could Kate say to herself to answer back to her negative thoughts about this situation? What would some more positive thoughts be?

Would thinking differently change her time at the party?

First Day at School

What you say to yourself can directly affect your feelings and behaviour. Your thoughts have huge power over your feelings.

Caitlin and Jacob are starting their first day of school. Caitlin thinks to herself, 'I am going to have the best day!! I can't wait to get there, I have my books all ready and I know the teacher is going to be really nice!!' On the other hand, Jacob says to himself, 'I don't really want to go; I know I'm not going to have a very good time. No-one will talk to me, I'm sure I'll get in trouble on the first day.'

What emotions would Caitlin be feeling? Why?

What emotions would Jacob be feeling? Why?

How would Caitlin behave at school? Would she be likely to have a good time?

How would Jacob behave at school? Would he be likely to have a good time?

What could Jacob say to himself to answer back to his unhappy thoughts about going to school? What could he say to cheer himself up?

Would thinking differently change his time at school?

Challenging your Thoughts

When you feel upset, angry, scared or sad, see if you can catch the thoughts behind those feelings. For example, if someone feels scared they could be thinking: 'Oh no! I'm sure something bad is going to happen!'

Once you have caught the unhelpful thoughts, use one of the challenges below:

- **Am I making a big deal out of this?**

- **Am I sure this is really going to happen?**

- **Does it really matter what other people think?**

- **Is this really true?**

- **Is it the end of the world?**

- **Have I coped with this before?**

- **Is it helping me to think like this?**

- **If my best friend thought this way, what would I say to them?**

- **How could I answer back to this thought to put it in its place?**

Changing your Thinking

Event: _____

Behaviour: _____

Emotions (0–10): _____

Thoughts What you actually told yourself	Challenge Pick a challenge question from the Challenging Your Thoughts list for each thought – answer back to your thought!	Alternative thought A more helpful and realistic thought
		How do you feel now? Emotions (0–10):

Helpful Thoughts, Unhelpful Thoughts

Some thoughts are unhelpful because they make you feel sad or scared, other thoughts are helpful because they make you feel happy and safe. When you have an unhelpful thought, see if you can turn it around into a helpful thought! Try below!

Unhelpful thoughts	Helpful thoughts
'Nobody likes me.' 'I'm bad because I got in trouble.'	'I have one good friend and I will make more.' 'I did one thing wrong, that doesn't make me a bad person.'

2.4 Emotional regulation

The worksheets in this section encourage children and adolescents to better understand their emotional reactions and the negative behaviours that often stem from them (e.g. tantrums, aggression, self-harm, substance abuse, eating issues). The exercises aim to increase the client's awareness of their emotions and behaviours and to put in place more adaptive responses.

Warning Sign

Suitable for: any age

This sheet focuses on one problem emotion in depth. It looks at how this emotion causes problems for the client and how they can detect it early in its development to prevent its escalation. Even very young children can draw their negative emotion and think about what happens in their body first when this emotion is 'visiting'. By tuning in to their early warning sign, young clients can become proficient in using mood management strategies.

Knock-on Effect

Suitable for: older children and adolescents

This exercise asks children and adolescents to think about the behavioural consequences of their unhelpful emotions. It guides them to reflect upon what happens when their problem emotion 'visits' them and the negative consequences of the behaviours they tend to engage in when emotional. The aim of this sheet is to encourage young clients to think about the consequences of their actions in order to motivate them to detect their emotion early (early warning sign) and to use an adaptive behavioural strategy, rather than letting the emotion run its usual course.

Feel-good Strategies

Suitable for: any age

This sheet is useful for the therapist and the client to brainstorm a list of strategies to help the client feel more positive should they experience prolonged negative emotions. It provides an opportunity for the therapist to emphasise the importance of adaptive behaviours in emotional self-regulation.

Licence to be Calm

Suitable for: children

This sheet contains an outline for a licence to be calm. This is to be completed, cut out and, if possible laminated so that it can have a string tied to it or a safety-pin stuck on the back, so that it can be worn by the child either around their neck or as a badge. There is space for the child to put their photo or to draw themselves, and space to list their calm strategies. This serves as a constant reminder of the things that they are licensed to do to remain calm and in control of their feelings. This is especially useful for young children and they must be highly praised whenever they use their licence.

Warning Sign

Which emotion causes the most problems for you? (name and draw it below)

How and why does this emotion cause you problems? How does it mess up your life?

What happens first in your body when this emotion is visiting you? (e.g. tense muscles, tight chest, heart pounding, sweating, sick in the stomach, want to cry, etc.)

THIS IS YOUR EARLY WARNING SIGN!!

Knock-on Effect

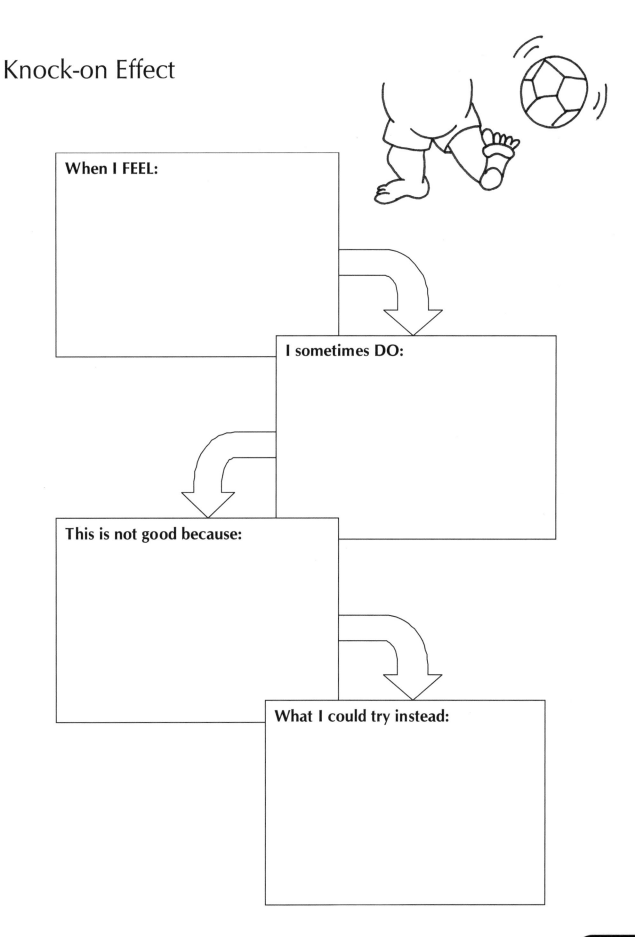

When I FEEL:

I sometimes DO:

This is not good because:

What I could try instead:

Feel-good Strategies

List some things you could do to cheer yourself up when you need to!

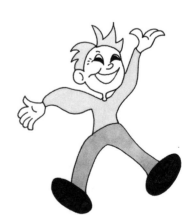

Licence to be Calm

Licence to be calm

Owner: _____

Calm strategies:

-
-
-

2.5 Goal-setting

This section concentrates on goal-setting by looking at what goals are and why we have them, how to set a goal, and ways to motivate your client to achieve their goals. The sheets are practical and self-explanatory but can greatly help the client to be motivated and focused throughout the therapy process. Most of the concepts in this section are best suited to older children and adolescents, but with younger children their parents/caregivers might benefit from using the sheets to look at the goals of therapy.

What is a Goal?

Suitable for: older children and adolescents

This is an information sheet about what goals are and how to set goals. It has room for older child or adolescent clients to think about some of their goals.

Goal-setting

Suitable for: older children and adolescents

This sheet guides the client through the process of goal-setting. It is a fairly detailed format for more complex goals and would be most appropriate for older children or highly motivated adolescents. This gives the therapist a chance to coach the client in good goal-setting habits. Once the client understands this process, this sheet can be a useful homework sheet to encourage the client to set, plan and monitor their own goals.

My Goals

Suitable for: any age

In this exercise, the client has room to plan four goals in less detail than the last sheet. This is likely to suit adolescents or children with less complex goals. It is a less threatening sheet that is quick and easy to use.

Goal for the Day, Goal for the Week

Suitable for: any age

This sheet asks clients to think of short-term and longer-term goals. Its simple format makes it non-threatening and ideal for sticking up on the wall to prompt continued work on the goals. It demonstrates to the client that in order to achieve their longer-term goals, they need to begin working on them each day. The focus on rewards provides an incentive to achieve the goals. This is especially important for children because the goal itself may not be intrinsically rewarding (i.e. keeping a tidy room), so the reward becomes vital in providing this encouragement.

In Five Years' Time...

Suitable for: older children and adolescents

This sheet is valuable for illustrating to young people that they need to begin working towards their long-term goals now. It encourages them to think about what is important to them and who they want to be in the future. It is important that the therapist validates their plans and helps them to break those plans (no matter how outlandish!) down into realistic, manageable steps to help them to begin. Obviously, this is best suited to older children and adolescents.

What is a Goal?

A goal is something that you want to achieve. Sometimes goals are easy and other times goals are very hard. Some examples of goals are:

- becoming a faster runner

- keeping a tidier room

- doing your chores

- doing your homework each night

- finishing reading a book

- getting to the next level of a computer game

- eating your vegetables.

How do you set goals?

1. NAME YOUR GOAL: think about WHAT it is that you want to achieve and WHY it is important.

2. Break your goal down into SMALL STEPS so that each step is a reasonable size.

3. THINK about your goal EVERY DAY and work towards it.

4. Set REWARDS that you can achieve as you work towards your goal.

What are some of your goals?

-

-

-

Goal-setting

My goal: _____

Why I want to achieve this goal: _____

_____

Step 1: _____

Step 2: _____

Step 3: _____

Step 4: _____

What do I need to achieve this goal (help, time, materials etc.)? _____

_____

What might make it hard to achieve this goal? _____

_____

Solutions to these problems: _____

_____

When would I like to have this goal achieved? _____

_____

My Goals

GOAL 1 _____

_____

Step 1: _____

_____

Step 2: _____

_____

Step 3: _____

_____

Step 4: _____

_____

GOAL 2 _____

_____

Step 1: _____

_____

Step 2: _____

_____

Step 3: _____

_____

Step 4: _____

_____

GOAL 3 _____

_____

Step 1: _____

_____

Step 2: _____

_____

Step 3: _____

_____

Step 4: _____

_____

GOAL 4 _____

_____

Step 1: _____

_____

Step 2: _____

_____

Step 3: _____

_____

Step 4: _____

_____

Goal for the Day

My goal for the **day** is: _____

_____

_____

_____

Reward for achieving this goal: _____

_____

_____

Goal for the Week

My goal for the **week** is: _____

_____

_____

_____

Reward for achieving this goal: _____

_____

_____

In Five Years' Time...

In five years' time I will be aged: _____

In five years' time I will be a person who:

_____

_____

_____

I will no longer be a person who:

_____

_____

_____

To reach these goals what do I need to start doing now?

_____

_____

_____

Who or what can help me reach these goals?

_____

_____

_____

2.6 Problem-solving

This section contains information on solving problems. This is most appropriate for older children and adolescents. The theory of problem-solving and the following exercises set a valuable foundation in problem-solving for young people to take into adulthood.

Thinking through a Problem

Suitable for: older children and adolescents

This first sheet is an exploratory sheet that gives older children or adolescents space to think a problem through in detail. It asks them to clarify what is bothering them and to think about why this is bothering them. It asks them to think about what they would like to happen in this situation and to reflect upon how likely this is. This sheet is helpful to pre-empt the following 'What to Do?' sheet for more structured problem-solving.

Solving Problems: What to Do?

Suitable for: older children and adolescents

This is a problem-solving sheet for children and young adolescents that guides them through the steps of problem-solving, using an example. It takes them through the theory of problem-solving by defining the problem, generating options and weighing up each before finally selecting and planning the best option. This serves as a guide for clients when they use the blank 'What to Do?' sheet with their own example.

What to Do?

Suitable for: older children and adolescents

This is a blank problem-solving sheet to allow the child or adolescent client to work through their own problem as they are guided through the steps of problem-solving. It could be a useful tool in therapy or as a homework task. For young children who are not reading and writing well, the therapist could talk them through the steps to model how to think about all the things they could do to solve a problem and to pick the best option. This provides an opportunity for modelling the skill and discussion about the problem in detail.

Introduce the parents/caregivers to this strategy, so that they can be sure to model its use, as well as giving children and adolescents time to work through a problem themselves without the caregiver solving it for them. This is important for developing young clients' sense of accomplishment and faith in their own coping ability when faced with problems.

Thinking through a Problem

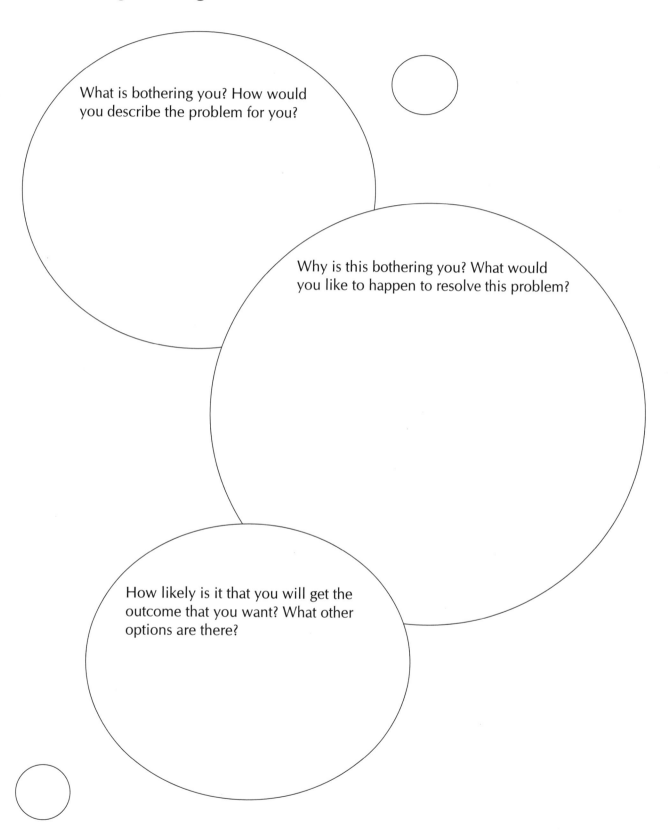

What is bothering you? How would you describe the problem for you?

Why is this bothering you? What would you like to happen to resolve this problem?

How likely is it that you will get the outcome that you want? What other options are there?

Solving Problems: What to Do?

Sometimes it is easier to solve a problem if you think it through first. Follow these steps to see if you can find a solution to John's problem.

1. What is the problem?
John really wants to go to his friend's house on Saturday but his parents can't drive him. He hasn't seen this friend in ages and really wants to go.

2. Make a big list on the back of this sheet of all the things you can think of to solve it. Then pick the best four and write them in below.

3. The best four options

Options	Good things	Bad things
Ask John's friend's parents to pick him up.	*John gets to see his friend.*	*His friend's parents might not want to pick him up.*
Get a bus.	*John gets to see his friend.* *No-one has to drive him.*	*Might not be allowed.* *Could be unsafe.* *Might not be a bus stop close.*
Get a taxi.	*John gets to see his friend.* *No parents have to drive him.*	*Could be costly.* *Might not be allowed.* *Could be unsafe.*
Arrange to see his friend next weekend.	*Doesn't cost anything.* *No parents have to drive him anywhere this weekend.*	*Will miss out on seeing his friend this weekend.*

4. Pick the best option! *Ask John's friend's parents to pick him up.*

5. Put it into action (*What would you need to do? What help would you need? When are you going to do it?*):

Call friend's parents as soon as possible and ask them if they would mind picking John up.

What to Do?

Sometimes it is easier to solve a problem if you think it through first. Follow these steps to see if you can find a solution to your problem.

1. What is the problem?

_____

_____

2. Make a big list on the back of this sheet of all the things you can think of to solve it. Then pick the best four and write them in below.

3. The best four options

Options	Good things	Bad things

4. Pick the best one!

5. Put it into action (What would you need to do? What help would you need? When are you going to do it?):

_____

_____

_____

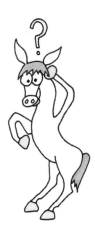

MAIN COURSE

SECTION 3 ANXIETY ISSUES

3.1 Psycho-education and increasing awareness

This section contains a basic psycho-educational handout about anxiety for the child or adolescent client, as well as some information sheets for the parent/caregiver of an anxious child or adolescent. For a more detailed and biological description of anxiety, panic attacks and phobias see the companion volume to this book *Gourmet Fast Food Handouts for Working with Adult Clients*. The exercises in this section also aim to increase young client's awareness of their anxiety to improve its early detection.

Feeling Scared

Suitable for: any age

This is an information sheet for children about anxiety. It uses simple language and pictures to explain what anxiety is and some of its physical symptoms. For very young children it could also be talked through with the therapist or parents.

Parents: Supporting your Anxious Child

Suitable for: any age

This is an information sheet for parents of children and adolescents who suffer from anxiety. It explains some of the different anxiety disorders and their symptoms. This may help parents to better understand their child's experience of anxiety and so reduce their confusion or frustration with their child's symptoms. It outlines what to look for in children, so that parents may be better able to detect and interpret the early warning signs of anxiety.

Parents: Aiding Treatment for Anxiety

Suitable for: any age

This is an information sheet for parents of children and adolescents who are undergoing treatment for anxiety disorders. It provides information on how best to support a child through the treatment of anxiety and gives specific suggestions for how parents can compliment and enhance their child's therapy.

Monitoring Anxiety

Suitable for: any age

This sheet instructs the client to monitor their anxiety throughout the day, first rating its severity out of 10, then recording their symptoms, and finally recording the events that were taking place at the time. It works by increasing the client's awareness of their environmental triggers and heightens recognition of their subjective levels of anxiety. This is mainly aimed at older children and adolescents, owing to its complexity, but it could be completed by the parents of a younger child to gather information about their child's anxiety. Parents of younger child clients could also use this sheet to encourage their child to rate their anxiety throughout the day, thus increasing their awareness.

Body Clues

Suitable for: any age

In this exercise, the client records their physical symptoms of anxiety onto the picture. This is very helpful for increasing children's and adolescents' awareness of the physical cues of anxiety so that they can more quickly detect its onset and can know when to use mood management strategies. There are two versions provided, one for males and one for females.

Feeling Scared

It is no fun feeling scared! But...

...it is normal to feel scared sometimes because this lets us know when something is not right.

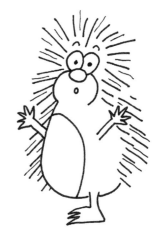

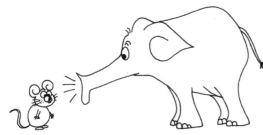

For some people, they feel scared a lot of the time and this makes them unhappy.

Do you ever feel scared?

You can feel scared in almost any part of your body:

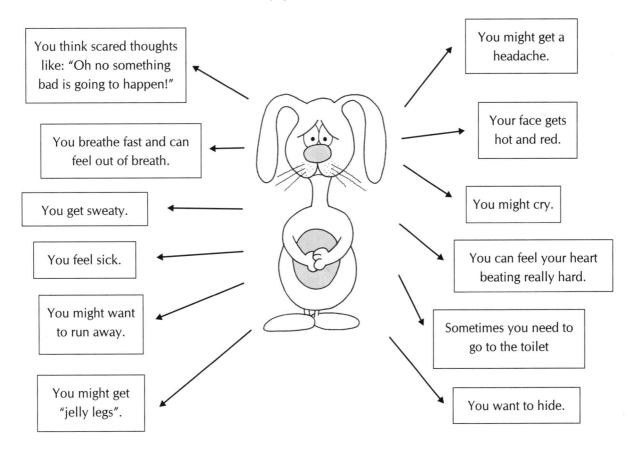

You think scared thoughts like: "Oh no something bad is going to happen!"

You breathe fast and can feel out of breath.

You get sweaty.

You feel sick.

You might want to run away.

You might get "jelly legs".

You might get a headache.

Your face gets hot and red.

You might cry.

You can feel your heart beating really hard.

Sometimes you need to go to the toilet

You want to hide.

Parents: Supporting your Anxious Child

What is anxiety?

Anxiety is a term that describes an emotional reaction to a perceived threat, and is often known as the 'fight/flight' response. This is an adaptive response designed to protect the individual from harm. When in real danger, anxiety and its accompanying cluster of physiological symptoms serve to promote our safety. However, when the anxiety reaction becomes overly sensitive, it can disrupt normal life and become extremely debilitating for the individual.

Detecting your child's anxiety

When children suffer from extreme anxiety, you may notice that they become preoccupied with worries and fears, that they have a range of physical concerns (nausea, tension, headaches, sweating, shaking, shallow breathing, rapid heart rate, etc.), and that they try to avoid particular situations (such as school, germs, social situations, crowds, the dark, being alone, or confined spaces). They may become tearful, prone to angry outbursts, begin to display oppositional behaviour, or become overly controlling.

Different types of childhood anxiety

Anxiety in children and young people can manifest in many different ways:

- **separation anxiety:** marked distress when separating from a caregiver or from home, worry about the safety of that person, and clingy behaviour with that person. This is often described as 'school refusal'.

- **panic disorder:** short-lived episodes of extreme anxiety, including extreme physical symptoms and a fear of dying or 'going crazy'. These attacks happen often and in a variety of situations.

- **generalised anxiety disorder:** a range of everyday worries that are out of proportion to the level of risk (e.g. worries over health, school work, the dark, intruders, significant others' safety) and impair functioning. Children often ask lots of 'what if?' questions.

- **phobias (including social phobia):** intense fear and avoidance of specific situations or objects (e.g. snakes, spiders, injections, social/performance situations). The fear and avoidance interfere with the child's life.

- **obsessive compulsive disorder:** extreme fears that cause significant anxiety and are accompanied by compulsive behaviours to reduce the anxiety (e.g. an extreme fear of getting sick prompts compulsive hand-washing to reduce the fear). The compulsions and rituals take over the child's life and serve to prolong their anxiety.

Parents: Aiding Treatment for Anxiety

Treatment for anxiety can be tough for anxious children and particularly difficult for their parents. It is important that parents understand how best to help their child through treatment so that they do not accidentally work against the treatment goals.

Helping your child through treatment for anxiety

The best thing a parent can do is to become knowledgeable about anxiety and to be aware of the specific mechanisms of their child's anxiety, including its triggers, the nature of the fears and what the child does to reduce their anxiety (such as avoidance, seeking reassurance, etc.). This will enable the parent to provide clear information to the therapist and to best apply the strategies of therapy.

Exposure therapy

Treatment for anxiety typically involves the client being prepared to face their fears in small steps while using anxiety management techniques, such as slow breathing, relaxation and positive thinking. Different therapists will use slightly different approaches to treating anxiety; however, an element of treatment will always involve challenging fears, and this may mean being uncomfortable and having to face something scary that has been avoided.

It is vital that parents are consistent and firm with anxious children and that they encourage them to face their fears. If parents allow children to avoid whatever it is that they are afraid of, this will actually make their anxiety worse. That said, parents need to take the advice of the therapist about how quickly children are expected to face their fears – *gradual* exposure is recommended; rushing children can lead to setbacks. Above all, parents need to be supportive and patient and give lots of rewards!

Accidental rewards

Parents need to be aware of accidental rewards for their child's anxious behaviour, such as receiving attention, getting out of difficult tasks, and providing endless reassurance. Where possible, the child needs to be encouraged to apply the strategies they are using in therapy and to manage their anxiety independently. Make specific rewards for 'brave' and independent behaviour.

Calm consistency

Parents need to be calm and consistent! They need to be aware of their own discomfort with their child's distress and be able to keep the long-term goals in mind, rather than giving in to the short-term desire to remove their child's immediate distress.

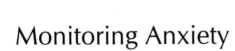

Monitoring Anxiety

Throughout the day, keep an eye on your anxiety by monitoring it (0–10), recording your anxious symptoms and what was happening at the time.

Time	Rate (0–10)	Symptoms	What was happening?
Early morning			
Mid-morning			
Lunch			
Afternoon			
Evening			

Comments:

_____

_____

_____

Body Clues

Draw or write onto the diagram all of the feelings and symptoms you experience when you are feeling **ANXIOUS** or **SCARED**.

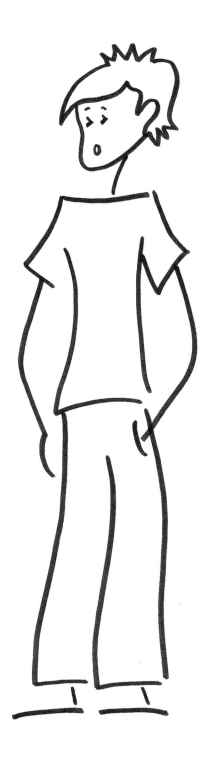

Body Clues

Draw or write onto the diagram all of the feelings and symptoms you experience when you are feeling **ANXIOUS** or **SCARED**.

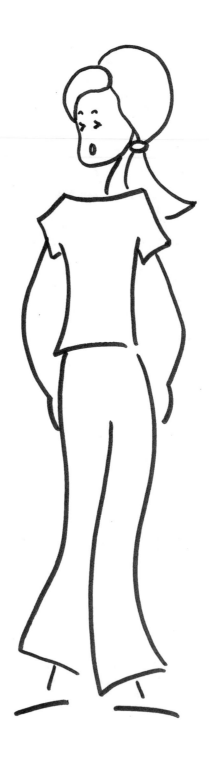

3.2 Anxiety reduction strategies

In this section, the young client is introduced to some different anxiety management strategies. Each strategy tackles anxious feelings from a slightly different angle in order to provide a range of activities to suit most age ranges and client presentations. It is always helpful for the therapist to teach the parent or caregiver the strategy as well as the client, so that they can coach them through the use of the strategy outside of therapy. Many parents can benefit from these strategies anyhow; so this benefits all!

Fire-breathing Dragon

Suitable for: children

This sheet teaches children how to use a slow breathing technique when they feel anxious. By giving the technique a fun but brave name, it inspires and empowers children to use it as a strategy for beating their anxiety. This strategy is most effective when applied early in the escalation of anxiety (i.e. as soon as the early-warning sign has been detected) and can significantly reduce the build-up of anxiety symptoms, thus giving the child a sense of control over their anxiety. For adolescents, the technique could be taught without the dragon analogy, using the 'in two three PAUSE – out two three' rhythm.

Slow Motion

Suitable for: any age

This is a brief technique that can be used to decrease the client's level of anxiety in the moment. It is not designed to solve the problem that is leading to the anxiety, it simply aims to help the client to manage at the time and reduce their levels of anxiety. It aims to improve the client's coping ability and confidence, to equip them for further exploration of their anxiety.

Slow Motion is most effective if the therapist practices the skill with the client in session, using real life examples, and gives them a card with the points of the skill on it to trigger their recall. The sheet has three 'slow motion' cards on it, so the therapist can copy them onto coloured card and perhaps laminate them, for distribution to their clients. If parents are coached in this technique, it can greatly increase its success. Some families may choose to enlarge the 'slow motion' card and stick it in a visible location in the house. This can then become a mood management technique used by all in the household.

Squeezing out Stress and Letting in Relaxation

Suitable for: any age

This is a progressive muscular relaxation script that the therapist could read out, accompanied by music in session, to train the child or adolescent client in an active relaxation technique. For younger children, a parent could read out the script so that they become familiar with the technique and can guide the child at home. This could be done before bedtime, in the car on the way to school, or played on a tape whenever needed by the young person. While useful for all anxious children, this technique can be particularly helpful for children who externalise their anxiety and tend to become angry or aggressive. This may be because it is an active form of relaxation that involves tension and release, thus helping them to diffuse tension actively.

Passive Relaxation Script

Suitable for: any age

This is similar to the above script, but this is a passive relaxation exercise that depicts a relaxing scene for the client to focus on while relaxing individual muscle groups. This example demonstrates the technique for clients, but could be substituted with any relaxing scene that helps the client to relax. As with the above script, the therapist could read out the script in session or instruct the client to read it out loud, while recording their voice onto tape so that they can use it as required. It could be an activity of therapy for the client to come up with their own relaxing and 'safe' place to imagine when they are feeling anxious and to put together a script for this.

Fire-breathing Dragon

When you feel scared or upset you can breathe like a FIRE-BREATHING DRAGON to feel more brave and strong!

To do this...

Step One

TAKE A DEEP BREATH...HOLD IT...AND COUNT TO FIVE:

1...2...3...4...5

...AND THEN BLOW IT ALL OUT LONG AND SLOW THROUGH YOUR NOSE...

LIKE

A FIRE-BREATHING DRAGON!

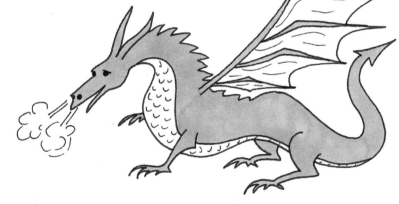

Step Two

NOW REPEAT BUT WITH SMALLER, SLOWER BREATHS!

COUNT: IN-TWO-THREE-PAUSE-OUT-TWO-THREE

Slow Motion

1. Monitor and name the emotion (0–10).

2. Look for your early warning sign.

3. **SLOW DOWN AND BREATHE:** abdominal breathing – 10 slow breaths.

4. Think calmly: **WHAT** is causing you to feel this way?

                            WHY is this upsetting you?

                            What can you **DO** to cope and reduce your feelings?

---

1. Monitor and name the emotion (0–10).

2. Look for your early warning sign.

3. **SLOW DOWN AND BREATHE:** abdominal breathing – 10 slow breaths.

4. Think calmly: **WHAT** is causing you to feel this way?

                            WHY is this upsetting you?

                            What can you **DO** to cope and reduce your feelings?

---

1. Monitor and name the emotion (0–10).

2. Look for your early warning sign.

3. **SLOW DOWN AND BREATHE:** abdominal breathing – 10 slow breaths.

4. Think calmly: **WHAT** is causing you to feel this way?

                            WHY is this upsetting you?

                            What can you **DO** to cope and reduce your feelings?

Squeezing out Stress and Letting in Relaxation

To help you to feel less stressed and more relaxed, we are going to do some exercises for you to squeeze out your stress and let in the nice calm feeling of relaxation. To do this, start by making sure that you are comfortable, that you are in a quiet place and that you are ready to relax.

Now, think about your feet. Imagine that you are knee-deep in wet sand at the beach and that you are digging down, down with your toes. Point your toes and tighten all the muscles in your feet...HOLD...pointing your toes...HOLD...and relax. Feel the warmth of relaxation seep into your feet, enjoy that feeling. Now, leaving the rest of your body relaxed...point your toes down hard again...HOLD...and release. Feel how nice and warm your feet feel when they are relaxed.

Now think about your legs. Still imagining that you are knee-deep in the wet sand at the beach, try to pull your legs out of the sand. Pull your legs up and tense them all up...HOLD that tension...harder...HOLD...and release. Feel how nice it is to relax your legs and let them go all floppy and soft. Now try and step out of the sand again, tense all your legs up hard...HOLD...HOLD...and release. Let all of the tension wash away through your toes with each outward breath. Feel how nice it is to have your whole legs and feet relaxed.

Now think about your stomach. Imagine that a HUGE boulder is about to be dropped on your stomach. It is really heavy! Tense and scrunch your stomach to protect it...HOLD...HOLD...and let go. Feel how good it is to relax your whole stomach. Oh no! Here comes the boulder again! Tense your stomach again...HOLD...that tension...HOLD...tighter...and release. Take a deep breath, in filling your whole chest...HOLD IT...and sigh it out, releasing all pent-up tension and resistance. Feel the warmth of relaxation filling every part of your stomach and trickling up your back.

Squeezing out Stress and Letting in Relaxation *cont.*

Now think about your shoulders and neck. Imagine that you are a turtle who has just got a big fright and you pull your head into your shell as tight as you can. Tense your whole neck and shoulders by pulling your head into your shoulders as far as you can...HOLD...HOLD...and relax. It seems that the turtle is not as scared now! Oh no! He has just seen something else that frightened him! Quick, pull your head back into your shell...HOLD...HOLD...and relax. Nothing to worry about, just enjoy feeling relaxed and soft in your whole legs, stomach, back and shoulders.

Next, think about your arms and hands. Imagine you are holding two rubbery stress balls and that you are squeezing them as hard as you can. Tense all the muscles of your hands and arms...HOLD...HOLD...and release. Let them become soft and floppy. Now squeeze those stress balls again, as hard as you can...HOLD...HOLD...and release. Let the tension flow out through your finger-tips and feel how nice it is to be relaxed.

Now, last, it is time to squeeze the tension out of your face. Tense the muscles of your face and neck by imagining that someone is trying to make you eat something that smells REALLY BAD! Clench your jaw tightly shut, close your eyes and scrunch up your whole face...HOLD...HOLD...and release. Let the relaxation melt into your face and jaw. Feel the relaxation, smoothing your face and releasing your jaw. Here they come again with the yucky food! Scrunch up your face and tighten your jaw...HOLD...HOLD...and release. Isn't it nice to relax rather than to be tense?

Now feel your whole body. Feel how relaxed and soft it is, no longer tense and uncomfortable. Remember what this feels like and do this whenever you feel tense and stressed.

Passive Relaxation Script

Start by sitting or lying in a comfortable position where your head is supported and your feet and legs are uncrossed. Now it is time to take a few moments to relax and get rid of any anxious, stressed or worried feelings.

Begin by thinking about your breathing. Make it smooth, slow and calm. Quiet your mind by concentrating on each and every breath. Your breath is like waves at the beach, washing gently and smoothly in and quietly slipping back out. Take a deep breath in and hold it...then sigh the breath out, releasing any worry, stress or tightness in your body. Your breathing is so easy. It soothes every corner of your body and makes you feel heavier and heavier. Make your breathing slower and slower as you relax more and more.

Imagine that you are lying on a beach and that as you relax more and more you sink a little deeper, so that the sand is moulded around your body, gently supporting you as you get heavier and heavier.

Feel the sun warm on your face. Think of your eyes, mouth, and forehead all relaxing and smoothing out. Let your tongue and jaw relax and feel warm and soft. RELAX... Let your face feel warm and free from tension. RELAX...

The sun begins to warm your shoulders and neck. It is warm and soothing, comforting and soothing away tension, letting it flow from your shoulders and neck out with each outward breath. Becoming soft and relaxed, warm and free of tension. Now the sun warms your arms and hands as well, warm and relaxed, feeling soft and loose, all tension flowing out with the help of the sun's warmth. All the muscles in your arms and hands are free of tension, no longer tight. No longer ready to move, just soft and loose. Your face, neck, shoulders, arms and hands are flooded with the warmth and relaxation of the sun.

The sun now begins to warm your stomach. Your breath flows in and out completely free of any stress or worry. Your belly is gently rising and falling as you breathe. Your whole body is relaxed and soft, filling with the warmth of the sun and the comfort of relaxation. All tension is released with each outward breath, flowing smoothly away, leaving only a feeling of calmness.

Passive Relaxation Script *cont.*

Now you roll over and the sun is warm on your back, soothing it and melting away tightness. Now the sun is warming and soothing your legs. They feel warm and heavy, sinking into the sand. Enjoy the feeling of complete relaxation, your whole body feeling soft and heavy and warm.

The warmth continues down to your feet, melting away the tightness, leaving total softness, calmness and peace. The tension is flowing out through your feet with each outward breath. Now your whole legs are relaxed, heavy and loose.

Feel your whole body relaxed, quiet and calm. Enjoy the feeling of relaxation from head to toe. Allow the feeling to wash over your whole body with each inward breath leaving you completely and totally relaxed.

As you relax on the beach, you can hear the sound of some birds...you can hear the water gently washing in and out and the quiet splashing of the waves. You can smell the salty smell of the sea and the sand and you can feel the soft sand underneath you and the warm sun on your skin. Enjoy this relaxation for a few moments.

Now become aware of your surroundings again, start to wriggle your fingers and toes, open your eyes, have a stretch if you like, and remember to keep the feeling of relaxation in mind whenever you feel tense, stressed or anxious.

3.3 Cognitive behavioural strategies for anxiety

This section provides some simple cognitive behavioural strategies for helping children to manage their anxiety. The first sheet explains exposure therapy to parents or caregivers so that they can assist with this process, and the following sheets are for completion by the child or adolescent client.

Exposure Therapy for Parents

Suitable for: any age

This is a psycho-educational sheet for parents or caregivers that provides a rationale for exposure therapy and its role in reducing anxiety. It is important that carers are informed about the treatment of anxiety disorders so that they do not inadvertently reinforce avoidant behaviours and contribute to the development of anxiety. This sheet describes graded exposure using a hierarchy, and how this can greatly help children to overcome their fears. Covering this material with parents ensures that they are fully informed about their child's treatment and are best able to contribute to the therapy process.

Beating my Fears in Small Steps

Suitable for: any age

This is an exposure therapy hierarchy sheet with steps for children to complete so that they can see how they are going towards their goal. This sheet does not focus on the repetition of the steps in the hierarchy because this can seem daunting for children. However, it should be explained to the child's parents that they will have to repeat each step until their child can feel more comfortable in that particular situation, before moving on to the next step. Rewards will be needed for each step to provide incentives for children to tolerate the discomfort of exposure therapy. It can be effective to have increasingly enticing rewards for each step to help the child to feel motivated to continue and to acknowledge the higher challenge of each step.

Parents need to be committed to this process and able to give rewards as soon as each step is achieved, so that the reward is paired with the goal achievement (for the generalisation of learning and operant conditioning).

Anxious Thoughts, Calm Thoughts

Suitable for: any age

This is a simple cognitive sheet for challenging anxious thinking patterns. This is useful for children or adolescents to teach them to catch their anxious thoughts and answer back to them in an uncomplicated format. The calm thoughts could be copied onto a small card that the client carries with them as a reminder of their more productive and calm thoughts. Alternatively, the helpful, calm thoughts could be put onto a poster to be read everyday.

Angel on my Shoulder

Suitable for: children

This sheet contains a picture of an angel. The purpose of this angel is to be a guardian angel who helps an anxious child to feel more brave and strong. The child is to record any brave or soothing thoughts onto or around their angel and to hang it above their bed or in another visible location. Reading the positive thoughts helps children to challenge their anxious thoughts and to be able to self-soothe.

This can be a highly effective technique for coping with nightmares, because children can look at their angel when they wake up at night and reassure themselves that they are alright. The angel can have reminders of using their breathing techniques and any other positive thoughts or images that help children to feel safe. If the page is blown up to A3 size there will be more room for the content.

Exposure Therapy for Parents

When a child or teenager is afraid of something, they will do all they can to AVOID it. This temporarily takes away their anxiety but actually leads to the growth of their anxiety in the long run because they never get a chance to prove their fears wrong.

Therefore, in order to reduce anxiety, therapy often focuses on 'exposure therapy' which means facing your fears. This is not easy – so the most manageable way to do this is by breaking the fear down into small steps and tackling each step one by one. This means that the child's confidence grows with each step and their fear weakens.

How do I support my child/teenager?

1. Understanding and motivation: Be very clear about what it is that your child is afraid of and why. Try to understand the fears behind their anxiety (no matter how irrational they seem) and try not to judge them for feeling anxious. Be very aware of all the different situations that trigger their anxiety and that they try to avoid.

2. Facing fears in small steps: With your therapist's help, break your child's fear down into small steps. This is most easily done by looking at all the situations that they avoid and breaking these down. Arrange these situations into order from the easiest to the hardest, and give them a rating out of ten for how anxious your child says they would be if confronted by that situation now. (Use the 'Feelings Thermometer' sheet on page 48 for this).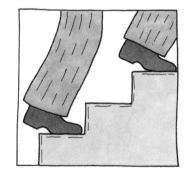

3. Start small, repeat each step: Set your child a goal of practising Step One several times over the next week. Make sure they stay in the situation long enough for their fear to decrease a little before stopping. Encourage them to use their helpful thinking strategies and their breathing techniques to help manage their anxiety. Repeat that same step over and over until they can do it with minimal anxiety.

4. Rewards: Each time your child completes a step of their exposure hierarchy they deserve a reward (for each practice) to provide an incentive. The prizes should get more meaningful as they progress through the plan. It is very important that the rewards are given straight after practice.

Beating my Fears in Small Steps

GOAL: _____

How scared this makes you (0–10)	FEARED SITUATIONS					
		REWARD				
			REWARD			
				REWARD		
					REWARD	
						REWARD

Anxious Thoughts, Calm Thoughts

Some thoughts make you feel anxious or scared, other thoughts make you feel calm and safe. When you have a scared thought, see if you can turn it around into a calm thought! Try below!

Anxious thoughts	Calm thoughts
'I can't do this.' *'What if something bad happens?'*	*'I have done it before and been fine, I can do it again.'* *'Nothing bad has ever happened before, I'll be OK.'*

Angel on my Shoulder

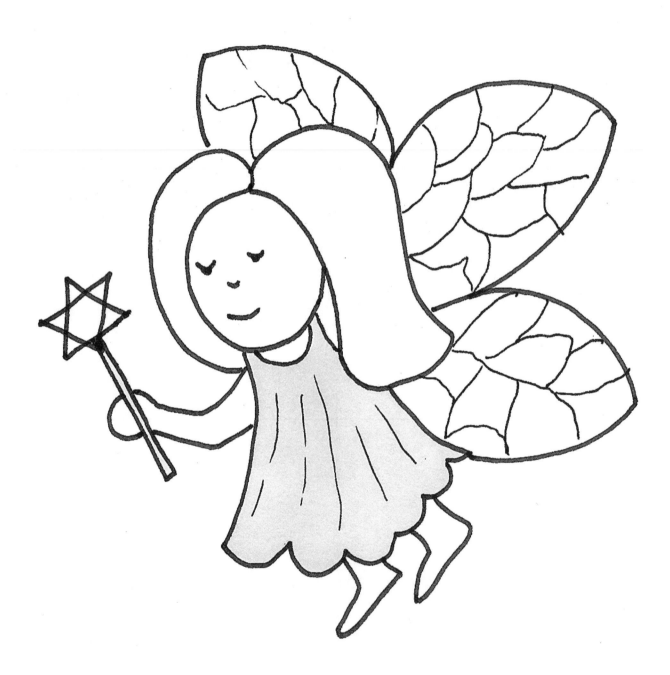

SECTION 4 DEPRESSIVE ISSUES

4.1 Psycho-education

These sheets are designed to give an introduction to the concept of depression for children and adolescents, as well as informing parents or caregivers about young people's reactions to depression and grief and loss. These strategies will complement worksheets from other sections of this book but are designed to target specific, depression-related symptomatology.

Why do I Feel so Sad?

Suitable for: children

This sheet aims to explain depression to children and young adolescents in a non-threatening manner. It uses animal pictures to represent the symptoms of depression for children. This might aid in their understanding of depression and be useful in generating discussion about the child's individual experience.

Sad Feelings

Suitable for: any age

This sheet encourages children and adolescents to identify the feelings and behaviours related to depression that they personally experience. It asks them to circle the feelings and behaviours that they experience when they feel sad or depressed. This allows the therapist to make an assessment about the level of the child's depression and the impact it is having on their life. This also opens up discussion about depression as a concept and can motivate the child to look at ways to beat it.

Grief and Loss for Parents

Suitable for: any age

This is an information sheet aimed at parents or caregivers to help them to understand the process of grief and loss in young people. It emphasises that grieving is an individual experience and that all people grieve in different ways. It intends to validate the child's experience of grief and to encourage parents to allow children to grieve in their own ways.

Why do I Feel so Sad?

Feeling sad some of
the time is normal...

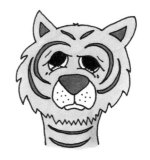

But for some people, they
feel sad all of the time.

Nothing seems to cheer
them up...

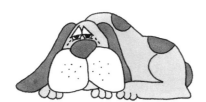

They have a lot of worries...

They want to hide away.

They cry a lot...

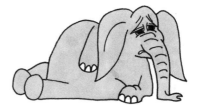

They get cranky...

They don't feel like
doing anything.

Do you ever feel like this?

Sad Feelings

Circle the things that you feel and do when you are sad...

Get in trouble a lot

Feel heavy

Cry

Can't laugh

Angry

Keep thinking
sad thoughts

Can't sleep

Cranky

Tired

Can't think

Scared

Headache

Sad

Worry

Don't feel like
doing anything

Yell and scream

Get a pain in
my tummy

Hide

Nothing's fun

Don't feel like
talking to
anyone

Stay in bed

Feel sick

Grief and Loss for Parents

There is no set response that children 'should' have or any predictable sequence that they will follow in their grieving experience. Children and young people often express their grief differently from adults, which can cause parents to worry that their child is not grieving appropriately.

Children may react to loss in the following ways.

DENIAL: children often do not comprehend what loss means, or cannot process such a large thing. This can lead to them trying to carry on as usual, but this often does not last. It is important that parents talk to the child about what the loss means, in a gentle manner.

ANGER: sometimes children can react to loss by becoming angry, oppositional and defiant. The anger they are expressing is a sign that they do not know how to make sense of what has happened and that they feel out of control. Children or teens who react in this way need support and understanding, someone impartial to talk to, and to be able to express their feelings in safe ways.

DESPAIR: some children express sadness, crying, hopelessness, and abandonment. Children reacting in this way may become anxious and clingy to loved ones and will need lots of reassurance and support. They need to know that it is OK to express their sadness, but that they have to live their life too.

GUILT: Some children may feel a sense of guilt, responsibility or blame for the loss. It is very important that these feelings are explored and challenged, so that they do not carry this burden unnecessarily.

ACCEPTANCE: Gradually, children will be able to accept the reality of the loss and to find some hope for the future.

Hints for dealing with grief

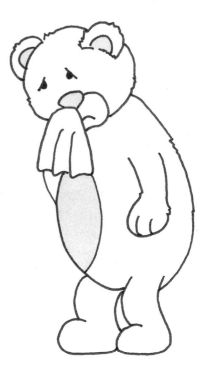

- Let children be involved in memory-making, such as making a collage or photo album, or planting a tree in memory of the loved one.

- Encourage children to release their feelings in healthy ways. Never discourage this.

- Support children with all that is familiar: people, places and surroundings.

- Allow yourself as the caregiver time to grieve as well. Do not be afraid to express some of your feelings to your child, so that they know that this is appropriate and part of healing.

4.2 Behavioural strategies for depression

This section contains activities to encourage children and adolescents to engage in pleasurable activities. These activities need to be planned in the same way that goals are planned and the parents/caregivers will need to be involved in this planning to ensure that pleasant activities can be carried out. This section also contains an exercise that guides older children and adolescents to think about the destructive things they engage in when depressed, and how to manage this.

Fun Things to Do

Suitable for: any age

This sheet provides a list of pleasant activities that can lift the mood of a depressed client. It provides an exhaustive list of options as well as serving as a visual prompt for pleasant activities. Additionally, it might help the therapist and client to discuss the importance of pleasant events in the recovery from depression. By doing something each day that is pleasurable, children's moods can be significantly lifted. These activities need not cost families a lot of money, but can shift a depressed client's focus from the negative to the positive.

Increasing Activity Levels

Suitable for: any age

This sheet explains the importance of pleasant activity in the treatment of depression and encourages the child or adolescent client to think of three activities they would like to do more of. The 'Fun Things to Do' list from the last sheet might serve as a prompt for this. Once the client has selected three activities, they could then use a sheet from Section 2.5, Goal-setting, to further plan this activity. Parents or caregivers will need to be included in this task so that they can ensure that appropriate selections are made and that the goals can be followed through.

Destructive Things I do when I am Down

Suitable for: adolescents

This exercise explores the activities that older children and adolescents might engage in when they are feeling depressed which can have a negative impact on their mood and their life. With the use of this sheet, these activities are brought up for discussion with the therapist and more helpful activities can then be generated. It allows for the discussion of destructive behaviours such as self-harm, aggression, withdrawal or substance abuse that clients might engage in when depressed. It could be used with younger children by simplifying the concept for them and by eliciting the help of their parents.

Fun Things to Do

Talking to a friend	Exercise/sport
Singing	Finishing something
Dancing	Getting dressed up
Listening to music	Being silly
Collecting things	Being with friends
Going for a holiday	Going to the movies
Setting goals	Making something from scratch
Relaxing	Talking to a friend on the phone
Having a long bath or shower	Listening to music
Swimming	Hobbies
Snorkelling	Repairing something
Patting your dog or cat	Giving someone a gift
Watching the sun set	Ice-skating or rollerblading
Being by the water	Walking
Listening to the sounds of nature	Drawing or painting
Going on a date	Lying in a peaceful place
Jogging	Arts and crafts
Smiling	Hugs
Calling a friend	Chocolate
Acknowledging what you have done well	Telling someone you love them
Lying in the sun	Doing absolutely nothing
Listening to others	Thinking about your own good qualities
Planning a party	Having breakfast in bed
Laughing	Sleeping
Telling jokes	Seeing a good movie
Reading	Doing something for someone else

Fun Things to Do *cont.*

Watching TV	Horseriding
Bushwalking	Sleeping in
Surfing	Gardening
Walking on the beach	Playing team sports
Staying up all night	Going for a drive
Eating your favourite meal	Flying a kite
Meeting new people	Afternoon nap
Going camping	Playing with a dog
Playing computer games	Playing a musical instrument
Diving into cool water	Hanging out with friends
Praying	Writing stories or poetry
Being with your family	Games with friends
Cleaning	Kicking a football
Sewing	Bike riding
Sightseeing	Exploring the internet
Going for a picnic	Cooking
Being pampered	Seeing live sport
Photography	Sailing
Fishing	Being alone
Writing in a diary or journal	Talking to a friend
Acting/drama	Meditating
Stargazing	Playing cards
Learning something new	Scrapbooking
Looking through photos	Having a hot chocolate
Lighting candles or incense	Going to museums or art galleries
Getting a massage	Going windowshopping
Going skiing	Believing that 'I'm OK.'

Increasing Activity Levels

To beat depression, you need to get active!
Think of three things that you like doing but that you haven't done for ages.
By doing these things, you take the first step to feeling better and beating depression.

What are two things you would like to do more of?

1. _____

Why? _____

How can you start this? _____

_____

2. _____

Why? _____

How can you start this? _____

_____

Destructive Things I do when I am Down

List in the left column some of the things you do when you are feeling down that have a negative impact on your life. Record what that negative impact is and then, in the right column, list some more helpful activities you could do to help you to feel a bit better.

Destructive things I do	Negative impact they have	More helpful things I could do

4.3 Cognitive strategies for depression

This section aims to add to the material already discussed in the Therapy Basics section, specifically in Section 2.3, Cognitive behavioural therapy. The techniques described here help to tailor cognitive therapy to the individual presenting predominantly with depressive issues. For more detailed cognitive work, particularly with older children and adolescents, see Section 2.3.

Happy Thoughts, Sad Thoughts

Suitable for: any age

This sheet is a simplified version of the 'Changing Your Thinking' sheet (on page 62) and is aimed at younger children to encourage them to acknowledge their sad thoughts and to try to replace them with happier, more positive thoughts. This will set up good habits in young children and pave the way for more in-depth cognitive work when they are older.

Positive Thinking Cue Cards

Suitable for: any age

These cue cards are designed to be used following a 'Changing Your Thinking' sheet (from page 62 in Section 2.3, Cognitive behavioural therapy) or the 'Happy Thoughts, Sad Thoughts' sheet above. The aim of this exercise is for the client to write down some realistic, positive thoughts onto a cue card so that they can refer to them regularly.

This aids in the learning of new patterns of thinking and serves as a reminder for the client of their new, more helpful ways of thinking. These cue cards could be laminated for the client to carry or made into posters or collages that they look at each day as they brush their teeth or get dressed in the morning. This will help the new, more helpful thoughts to become habit.

Happy Thoughts, Sad Thoughts

Some thoughts are unhelpful because they make you feel sad or scared, other thoughts are helpful because they make you feel happy and safe. When you have a sad thought, see if you can turn it around into a happy thought! Try below!

Sad thoughts	Happy thoughts
'Nobody likes me.' 'I'm bad because I got in trouble.'	'I have one good friend and I will make more.' 'I did one thing wrong, that doesn't make me a bad person.'

Positive Thinking Cue Cards

Positive thoughts

1. _____

_____

2: _____

_____

3. _____

_____

4. _____

_____

Positive thoughts

1. _____

_____

2: _____

_____

3. _____

_____

4. _____

_____

Positive thoughts

1. _____

_____

2: _____

_____

3. _____

_____

4. _____

_____

Positive thoughts

1. _____

_____

2: _____

_____

3. _____

_____

4. _____

_____

SECTION 5 ANGER ISSUES

5.1 Psycho-education

The exercises in this section explore anger as an emotion and aim to increase young clients' awareness and understanding of their anger. Some of the sheets are best suited to older children and adolescents because they contain more detailed concepts. Others are especially designed for younger children to help them to understand and label their experience of anger.

What Makes me Angry?

Suitable for: older children and adolescents

This is a psycho-educational and self-exploratory sheet for use with adolescents and older children. It encourages them to think about the things that make them feel angry and the symptoms they experience when angry. This may give insights into the triggers for anger and the client's general reaction to their anger.

Types of Anger

Suitable for: older children and adolescents

This is a psycho-educational sheet that describes some of the different ways that people express and deal with their anger. This aims to familiarise clients and their parents/caregivers with the many forms of anger, and to help increase their insight into their own methods of expressing their anger.

Symptoms of Anger

Suitable for: any age

This is a worksheet that asks clients to record their physical symptoms of anger. This will enable them to identify their anger symptoms, with a view to catching anger early and reducing it with some of the strategies listed in the Anger Management section (Section 5.3).

Anger Monster

Suitable for: children

This sheet is for use with children and uses a narrative style of questioning about anger. It guides the child to see their anger as an entity separate from themselves, which makes it easier for them to accept and deal with the problems that arise from anger. This follows on from the 'Narrative Therapy Questions' sheet on page 28 in Section 1.2, Boundaries and goals for therapy.

This is especially useful for children who feel that they are 'bad' for being angry. It positions the child in opposition to their anger, which can motivate them to fight back against it. This then provides an excellent platform for CBT and other behavioural interventions. Additionally, this approach aligns the therapist and client in their 'mission' against anger.

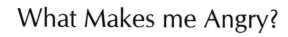

What Makes me Angry?

How do you know when you are angry? What happens in your body?

What sorts of things make you feel angry?

Why do these things bother you?

What would need to change in your life to reduce your anger?

Types of Anger

All people express anger in their own way. Anger can take many forms, below are some for the many ways that anger can be experienced.

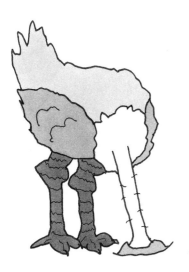

HEAD IN THE SAND

Some people find anger frightening. They shy away from acknowledging or expressing angry feelings and instead, convince themselves that they are *not angry*. The problem with this is that they do not release and express their feelings, which can lead to a build-up of frustration and unhappiness.

> *'I'm fine, I'm not angry at all.'*
> *'I don't mind.'*

RETREATING TO THE CAVE

Other people find anger so difficult to deal with that they do all that they can to *avoid* it. They try to hide in their 'cave' whenever they feel angry or whenever people around them are angry. Unfortunately, this means that they do not learn to manage their anger or other people's anger.

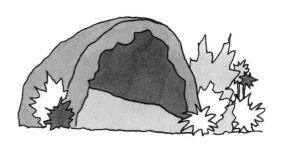

> *'I can't deal with this right now.'*
> *'Let's all just be friends.'*
> *'I don't want to talk about it.'*

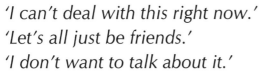

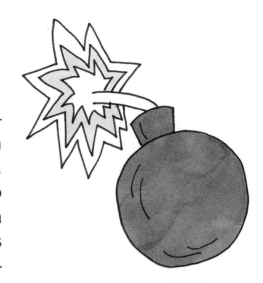

BOTTLERS

Some people find it very hard and very frightening to express their angry feelings, so they push them away and *hold onto* them deep inside. This can be because they fear getting into trouble or because they don't want to have a fight. Either way, bottling up angry feelings is like a ticking bomb that can lead to big explosions over little things down the track.

'I can't say anything because it will cause a fight.'
'I'll get into trouble if I say anything.'
'I'm not allowed to be angry.'

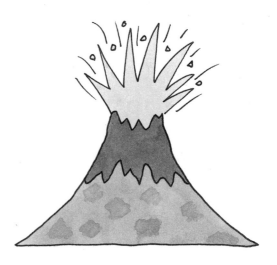

EXPLODERS

Some people yell and scream and 'blow off steam' when they are angry. They explode, lashing out at others either verbally or physically. This can provide a satisfying *release* for them in the short term, but can have bad consequences in the long term for themselves and their relationships.

'You stupid #@$%!'
'I'm right; everyone else is in the wrong and deserves to pay!'

Symptoms of Anger

Draw onto the bear all of the things that happen in your body when you feel angry.

Next, list around the picture some of the things that make you feel angry.

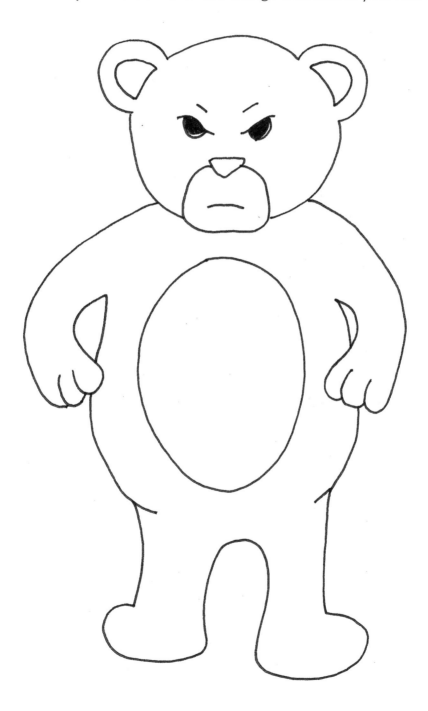

Anger Monster

Suzy is often visited by her ANGER MONSTER. She calls him 'Cranky-pants' because he makes her feel cranky, yell at others, and get into trouble. She knows when he is visiting her because her face gets hot, she feels sick in her belly, and she gets really tense in her arms and hands.

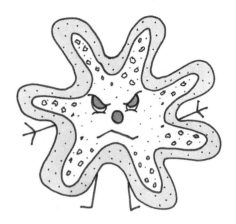

Do you have an ANGER MONSTER that visits you?

What is your monster's name? _____

How do you know when _____ **is visiting you?**

What changes happen in your body? _____

_____

How does _____ **make you feel?**

_____

What does _____ **make you do?**

_____

What is your life like when _____ **is in it?**

_____

_____

5.2 Motivation for managing anger

The following sheets help the client and therapist to further explore anger, its triggers, and how they deal with their angry feelings. This allows for monitoring of anger levels and close assessment of how the client and their caregivers respond to their anger. These exercises also give more information about triggers for anger and fears surrounding anger and its expression.

Monitoring and Exploring Anger

Suitable for: any age

This is a detailed monitoring sheet that could be completed by adolescents or the parents of children. It provides a wealth of information about the triggers for anger and how the client and their family react to their anger. This will provide a useful baseline for treatment so that progress can be measured and celebrated.

What I do with my Anger

Suitable for: older children and adolescents

This sheet aims to help clients to explore their particular method of managing their anger. It asks them what they would *like* to do (but never do) when they are angry, and to investigate why there is a difference between what they want to do and actually do with their anger. Some common roadblocks to releasing anger are then listed for the client to reflect on and to discuss with their therapist. This is particularly useful for adolescents who bottle, avoid or deny their anger. The concepts are probably a little complex for younger children.

Five Things that Make me Angry

Suitable for: any age

This is a sheet for children to help them to become aware of the different triggers for their anger. It asks them to list five things that they have an angry response to down the left column, and to describe what they do in the right column. This could be completed by a parent as a homework task or discussed with the child in session as a reflective tool. This is a more simplistic sheet that would suit younger children better than adolescents.

Monitoring and Exploring Anger

Anytime you feel angry (no matter how much or how little), record what happened in the table below:

What happened? Rate your anger (0–10)	Why did this make you feel angry?	What thoughts went through your mind?	What did you do (good or bad)?	Did these actions make you feel better or worse?

What I do with my Anger

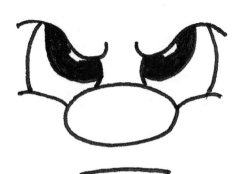

What I feel like doing when I am angry is:

-
-
-
-

What I actually do when I feel angry is:

-
-
-
-

Why is there a difference between what you would like to do and what you actually do when you are angry?

Copyright © Clare Rosoman 2008

Read through this list of roadblocks to releasing anger and tick those that apply to you:

- fear of hurting others (emotionally or physically)

- fear of ruining relationships

- fear of conflict

- feeling that anger is uncomfortable and unpleasant

- believing that you 'shouldn't' be angry

- worry that you will be judged for being angry

- feeling that you might lose control if you release your anger

- believing that anger is a weakness

- feeling that you should be able to 'deal with it' and stay calm

- believing that 'nice' people don't get angry

- fear that others will reject you if you are angry

- fear of the feeling of being angry – scary, unattractive, negative.

Five Things that Make me Angry

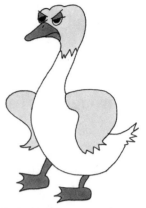

Something that makes me feel angry is...	How my body feels and what I do...

5.3 Anger Management

The sheets in this section provide some practical strategies for helping children and adolescent clients to manage their anger. They include several different strategies for immediate reduction of anger that might suit a varied range of clients.

Ready, Steady, GO!

Suitable for: any age

This is a simple technique for slowing down the escalation of anger into harmful behaviours. It involves the client in learning to identify their early warning signs of anger and being *ready* to engage in a more helpful, calming strategy (such as breathing, counting to 10, taking time out, going to a calm place, etc.). The second step is to be *steady* and to pause and notice the role of thinking in fuelling the anger. It is important for the client to tell themselves some calm thoughts at this time and to focus purely on how to stop their anger from escalating. The final step involves thinking about what actions they need to take to help the situation to resolve or to prevent further escalation of their anger.

This sheet provides the client with the steps for using this technique but it is important that the therapist go through the steps with them and coach them specifically in how to use it. Individual strategies (e.g. slow breathing) and examples of calming thoughts can be generated by the client and therapist and put on the sheet for the client to refer to. It is helpful if parents are involved in this process so that they can take on a coaching role with this technique.

Beating your Anger Monster

Suitable for: children

This sheet builds upon the 'Anger Monster' sheet on page 128 and is designed for children. It asks the child client to think about the ways that their anger 'ruins' their life and how to stop it from taking control. It continues to use the narrative style of questioning to help the child to oppose their anger and to feel motivated to try some anger management strategies as part of an armoury against their 'anger monster'.

It can help to have rewards for the child for attempting to go against their monster (by taking any steps to remain calm in situations that would normally trigger anger), and prizes that can be earned. If the therapist and family can monitor who is winning (i.e. the child or the monster) and award points and prizes (but not punishments for the child!), then the child's motivation to challenge their anger will continue to increase.

Staying Cool

Suitable for: any age

This is a list of simple anger management and distraction activities that could be used by children or adolescents when they detect their early warning sign that they are becoming angry. These techniques could give children ideas for beating their anger monster.

Ready, Steady, GO!

What is the first warning sign that you notice that lets you know that you are getting angry? *(usually something in your body – hot face, tense arms, sick in the stomach)*

When you notice this warning sign you need to **ACT FAST**:

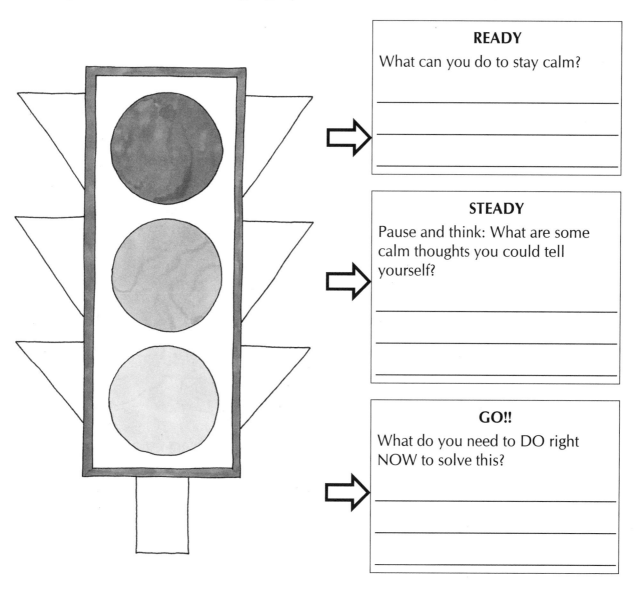

READY

What can you do to stay calm?

_____

_____

_____

STEADY

Pause and think: What are some calm thoughts you could tell yourself?

_____

_____

_____

GO!!

What do you need to DO right NOW to solve this?

_____

_____

_____

Beating your Anger Monster

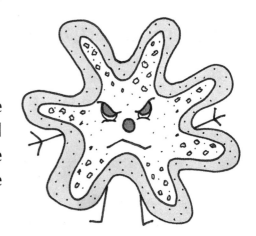

Suzy is often visited by her ANGER MONSTER. She calls him 'Cranky-pants' because he makes her feel cranky, yell at others, and get into trouble. She would like her anger monster to go away because he causes lots of problems for her and ruins her day.

Would you like to make your ANGER MONSTER go away? _____

What is your monster's name? _____

_____

How does _____ mess up your life?

What does _____ **make you do?**

- _____
- _____
- _____
- _____

Have you ever fought back? How?

_____

Can you think of some other ways to tell your monster to go away?

_____

How could you make him weaker than you?

_____

Are there any things that you can do to go against what he wants you to do? *(For instance, if he wants you to yell at the teacher, you could fight back by speaking calmly.)*

_____

Staying Cool

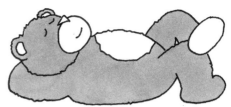

Staying cool when you feel angry can be HARD!
Here are some ideas to help you to stay in control
when you feel like getting angry.

Don't let your anger
have control over you.

Count backwards
from 10.

Take 5 slow deep
breaths.

Talk to a
friend about
what made
you angry.

Tell yourself calm things
like: 'It will be OK'

'It's not worth getting
angry over this'.

Get your mind off your
anger by doing
something else.

Be alone
for a while.

Write down your
feelings.

Make a quiet, safe
space somewhere in
your house and put calm
things in it, like books
and pictures
you like and a big
cushion to lie on.

Remember that you can
be stronger than your
anger.

Do
something
FUN.

Go there whenever
you feel you need to
be calm and relax.

6 COMMUNICATION SKILLS

6.1 Friendships

These sheets aim to help children and adolescents to explore their interpersonal relationships and to recognise when a relationship is healthy and when it is not. Some younger children may need to be guided through the exercises, but all the sheets raise important issues for discussion about communication and interaction with others for children and adolescents of all ages.

Friendships

Suitable for: older children and adolescents

This sheet asks children to think about their friendships. It first asks them what they look for in a friend and what they themselves have to offer friends. It then encourages them to reflect upon their friendships (this could be many if they are an adolescent!) and the different types of friendships they have. This can lead to meaningful discussion about expectations they have of certain friendships and the balance between input and output in some friendships.

Making Friends

Suitable for: children

A lot of children struggle to make meaningful friendships as a result of difficulty with social skills. This sheet asks the child to think about how to approach potential friends, show interest in others and make conversation with them. It also asks the child to think about how they could take a friendship from a superficial level to a deeper level (e.g. by inviting a friend over after school, by showing interest in them).

Promoting Healthy Friendships

Suitable for: older children and adolescents

This is a tip sheet listing some guidelines for healthy friendships and how to be a good friend. This might be useful to discuss with a client who is having difficulty in this area. It could open up discussion about past friendships and previous hurts.

Levels of Friendship

Suitable for: older children and adolescents

This sheet asks the client to write in all their friendships in relation to how close they feel to each person. This is a useful tool for the therapist to determine the level of social interaction and support available to the child. Further, discussion about this might develop the child's concept of boundaries and distance between themselves and others in their life.

What you Want from your Friends

Suitable for: older children and adolescents

This sheet generates ideas about the expectations of friendships. It asks the child to think about what they expect from their friends and what their friends expect from them in return. This might help the therapist to identify the client's needs within their friendships and any imbalances that might exist in their interpersonal relationships. This is particularly important for adolescent girls because their early girl–girl friendships often set the scene for their later romantic relationships.

When a Friendship is Unhealthy

Suitable for: older children and adolescents

This exercise encourages children and adolescents to really look at their friendships. If they have noticed that a friendship in their life is unhealthy, this sheet asks them to think about whether they want to save the friendship. If they do want to save it, they are encouraged to examine whether that friendship is unhealthy because of their own issues or owing to the other party. It then shows them how to construct an assertive message to voice their concerns. This could be discussed and practised with the therapist.

The value of this sheet is that it teaches the child or adolescent how to think critically about their relationships and their role in them. It encourages them to place importance on their own happiness in their friendships and explains that they do not have to keep unhealthy friendships in their life.

Peer Groups

Suitable for: adolescents

This sheet raises the concept of peer groups. The questions on this sheet might help the therapist to identify any unhealthy patterns within the adolescent client's peer group and the level of their attachment to the group. It is important that the therapist is never critical of the peer group but supportive of the young person's needs, gently questioning them about the health of their peer group and their satisfaction with it.

Resisting Pressure

Suitable for: adolescents

This sheet discusses the powerful desire to please friends that can sometimes lead children and adolescents into doing things they ordinarily wouldn't do. It then encourages the client to think of ways to say 'no' to resist future pressure. This sheet is useful for vulnerable young people who identify that they are easily swayed.

Scenarios for Resisting Peer Pressure

Suitable for: adolescents

This sheet contains several scenarios for discussion or role-play with the therapist to practise saying no and resisting the pressure of the peer group. Not all the scenarios will apply to all young people, but almost certainly some will resonate with them.

Coping with Exclusion

Suitable for: older children and adolescents

Exclusion is a difficult issue that commonly affects girls but can also happen to boys. Exclusion from the peer group is a very painful and threatening experience for a child or adolescent and is often used as a form of control and relational aggression among the peer group. This tip sheet lists some strategies for coping with exclusion that can be discussed and role-played in therapy, or given to the child to read through for homework.

Boys and Girls

Suitable for: older children and adolescents

This question sheet asks children and adolescents about their opinions about boys and girls and the differences in their relationships. This is a valuable tool for discussing boy–girl friendships with early adolescents who may be beginning to have boyfriends or girlfriends. It opens up discussion about these relationships, allowing the therapist to raise issues such as the benefits of having opposite-sex friends and healthy expectations for early romantic relationships.

Relationships

Suitable for: adolescents

This sheet explores the concept of romantic relationships compared to friendships. This can lead to open discussions about the difference between opposite-sex friends and a boyfriend or girlfriend, and the different roles and expectations of both. This is especially important to discuss with teens who may be beginning or are currently in a romantic relationship. Discussion about sexual behaviour and boundaries and resisting pressure might be highly valuable at this time.

Friendships

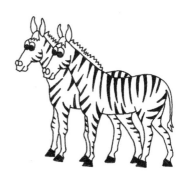

Describe the qualities you look for in a friend:

What qualities do you bring to your friendships?

Types of Friendships

In the boxes below, list some of your friends. Think about how your friendship with each is unique. Think about the strengths and weaknesses of each relationship.

Friends who you go to when you have a problem:	Friends you share a common interest with:	Someone who helps you to be a better person and to achieve your goals:
Friends who you only talk to sometimes:	Friends who you don't talk about problems with:	Friends who are just good fun:
Friends who share their problems with you:	Friends you can't trust with secrets:	Do you have any other types of friends? List them here:

Making Friends

Alistair has just joined a new school. What could he do to make new friends?

As he walks into the new classroom, what could he do with his body and face to show the other kids that he is a friendly person?

At lunchtime, he walks out into the playground and sees a group of kids from his class. What could he do to show them that he would like to get to know them?

What are some things he could talk to his new friends about?

Now that he has started talking to them, what could he do to become better friends with them?

Promoting Healthy Friendships

Friendships are important to all people. However, they take work and ongoing maintenance for them to stay healthy. To keep your friendships healthy try to:

- listen to your friends' needs

- be honest about your feelings with your friends

- don't intentionally try to hurt their feelings

- be prepared to say sorry when you make a mistake

- don't say sorry when you don't mean it

- don't say bad things about your friends to others, even when you are angry at them

- remember that no-one is perfect and we all make mistakes

- forgive your friends when they say sorry

- if someone else is saying bad things about one of your friends, tell them that you don't want to hear anything bad said about any of your friends and walk away. Don't join in

- accept differences in others

- don't expect one friendship to meet all your needs

- try to build lots of different friendships from different areas of your life

- allow your friends to have other close friends without getting jealous; remember that all people need lots of different types of friendships

- allow your friends to have different opinions to you

- don't feel you have to be exactly the same as your friends; individuality makes friendships interesting and exciting

- don't tolerate bad treatment from your friends, if they repeatedly hurt your feelings or break your trust, these are signs that your friendship is unhealthy and you might need to pull away a bit to protect yourself

- keep your friend's secrets (unless you think an adult really needs to know about it).

Levels of Friendship

Write in all the people in your life, showing how far away or close to you they are.
That means how close you feel to them emotionally.

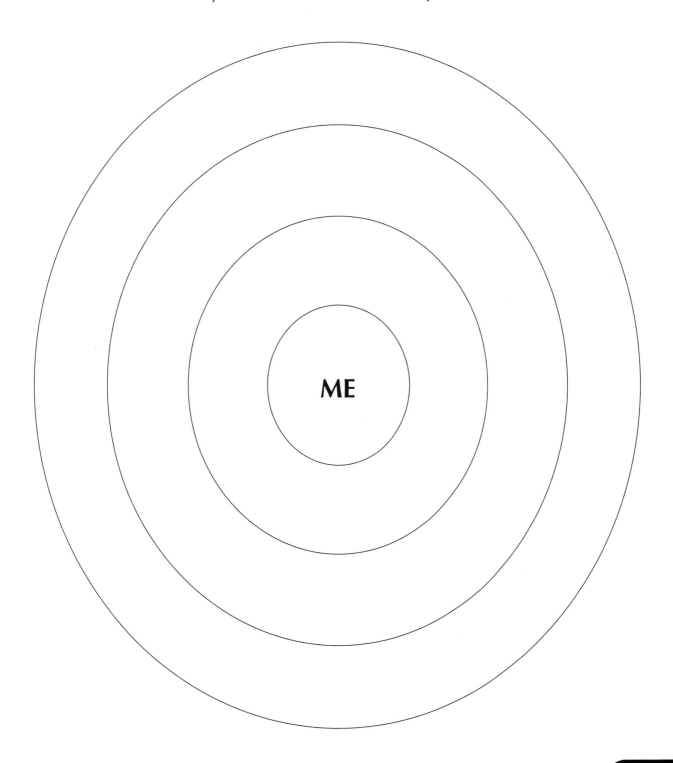

What you Want from your Friends

The following questions ask you to think about your friendships and to really look at what you expect of your friends (e.g. to keep your secrets, to listen to your problems) and what they expect of you (e.g. to be loyal to them, to sit with them in class).

What do your friends expect of you in your friendship with them?

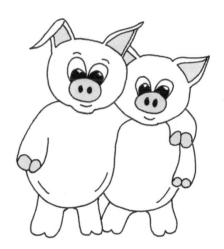

What do you expect of your friends?

Are there any differences between what you expect of them and what they expect of you?

Are your rights ever violated in your friendships? If they are, how? What have you tried to do about this?

When a Friendship is Unhealthy

What do you do when you know something is not right in a friendship? First, you need to think things through:

What is unhealthy in this relationship? What upsets you the most?	What solutions can you think of?	Is the friendship worth saving? What needs to change?

If you want to save a friendship, you need to look at **what needs to change** and decide whether it is something **you** need to change within you (how you communicate with the other, what you expect of the other), or whether the **other person** needs to change in how they deal with you.

If the other person needs to change, you have to tell them that in an open, sensitive and caring way (not blaming or criticising them). Try it like this:

I feel _____ (your emotion: *upset, left out, sad, etc.*)

When you _____ (what they **do**: *don't invite me places, ignore me*)

I would like _____ (what you want them to **do** differently: *include me*)

When a Friendship is Unhealthy *cont.*

Try these examples:
1. Anna feels pressured by Kara to not like Suzy. What could she say to Kara?

I feel _____

When you _____

I would like _____

2. Sam wasn't invited to Andrews's birthday party when the rest of their group was. What could Sam say to Andrew?

I felt _____

When you _____

I would like _____

Now try your own for the friendship problem you wrote about in the table. Practice saying it, ask for advice, then pick the right time and say it!!

I felt _____

When you _____

I would like _____

Peer Groups

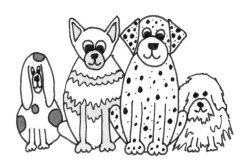

What is your peer group like? Who is in it? *(Draw below.)*

Do you have several different peer groups? List them...

Do you try not to let your friends down? What would happen if you did?

Are there any rules for membership to your group? What happens if someone does the wrong thing?

What would you do if you noticed that you were wearing different clothes from your friends or they wanted to do something that you didn't?

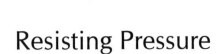

Resisting Pressure

Sometimes people feel under pressure to be a certain way to fit into a group. This can mean that you go against who you are and your values (*rules you live your life by, e.g. I don't like to say bad things about people, I am trustworthy, I don't steal*). You will know that you are going against your values if you feel guilty, reluctant or disappointed with yourself. If this happens you can say no – it just takes practice!

Can you think of a time when you did something that you didn't want to do but you did it anyway because your friends were?

_____

_____

_____

_____

How could you have handled that situation better?

_____

_____

_____

_____

Some different ways I can say 'no':

_____

_____

_____

_____

Scenarios for Resisting Peer Pressure

Scenario 1

A friend has borrowed some CDs and returned them scratched. You have just bought another CD and it is your favourite and they ask to borrow it. Write an assertive response.

Scenario 2

A friend offers you a cigarette and you don't want it. Write an assertive response.

Scenario 3

One of your friends decides they don't like another person in the group (that you do like) and that they don't want you to talk to that person anymore. Write an assertive response.

Scenario 4

Some of your friends are going to skip maths class by saying they're going to the toilet, but they plan to meet up elsewhere. They ask you to join in but you don't want to. Write an assertive response.

Scenario 5

Your friend wants to lie to their parents by saying they will be at your house when really they are going to a party with people from an older grade. They want you to tell their mum that they are at your house. Write an assertive response.

Coping with Exclusion

It is hard enough making friends, but what do you do when others try to exclude you? How do you cope when those who you once called friends are now the ones who try to keep you out?

---

1. Your first step has to be detachment!

You have to really stop caring that others don't want to include you. This is incredibly difficult but essential. It is important for two reasons; first, if you care too much, there can be damage to your self-esteem, and second, while you still react or come across as hurt, the people who want to hurt you will know that they have got to you.

By detaching and giving off an attitude of *'No matter what you say, I am worthwhile and I am comfortable and happy!'* you will have won half the battle. Never give them the thrill of knowing they have upset you, and they will probably get bored and find something else that interests them.

---

2. Step back and seek out others.

You can do this through activities; get involved in activities both inside and outside of school. Do something to keep yourself active and occupied. You'll care less about being excluded if you are too busy to think about it! Also, when you get involved in new activities, you are going to meet new people. If your exclusion is limited to an old group of ex-friends, you'll be sure to find new friends this way. Get involved with others and others will get involved with you!

---

3. Remember no-one has the right to bully or intimidate you. If you feel that others are purposely trying to hurt you, saying mean things, or doing anything else that makes you uncomfortable, you should talk to someone at school or at home who can put a stop to it.

Boys and Girls

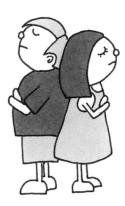

1.   Boys annoy me when _____

     _____

2.   What is important to girls in a relationship is _____

     _____

3.   It's good to be a boy because _____

     _____

4.   Parents would like girls to _____

     _____

5.   Parents would like boys to _____

     _____

6.   Boys get embarrassed when _____

     _____

7.   Boys don't understand girls because _____

     _____

8.   Girls cry when _____

     _____

Boys and Girls *cont.*

9.   Girls annoy me when _____

_____

10.   What is important to boys in a relationship is _____

_____

11.   Boys cry when   _____

_____

12.   It's good to be a girl because _____

_____

13.   Girls get embarrassed when _____

_____

14.   Girls don't understand boys because _____

_____

Relationships

What is the difference between a close friend and a boyfriend/girlfriend?

What is important when choosing a boyfriend/girlfriend?

Should your boyfriend/girlfriend be like a best friend? Why?

Should you share similar interests with your girlfriend/boyfriend? Have similar personalities? Why?

6.2 Assertiveness

In this section, children and adolescent clients are introduced to some key concepts of communication. First, the worksheets focus on assertiveness and different communication styles. Second, the exercises move on to specific communication skills to improve assertiveness. Finally, we look at dealing with conflict. The assertiveness and communication skills in this section use child-focused language and examples to aid in their understanding of the skills and how to apply them to their life.

Fight–Flight

Suitable for: older children and adolescents

This activity uses an easy and non-threatening questionnaire to determine the child's approach to communication. The items in the questionnaire provide interesting information for the therapist to discuss with the client about communication, as well as highlighting their individual style. This exercise increases the client's insight into their own interpersonal style (whether they are prone to fight or to flight).

Assertiveness

Suitable for: older children and adolescents

This sheet explains the concept of assertiveness and its benefits. It also presents some suggestions for increasing assertive behaviour that could be discussed and practised in therapy. Assertive skills such as 'I' statements are explained and examples given.

Saying 'NO'

Suitable for: older children and adolescents

This sheet provides the child or adolescent client with many examples for how to say 'no', should they need to. This is especially important for clients who succumb to peer pressure. It is helpful for the therapist to role-play with the client so that they become accomplished in this skill before having to use it in a real life situation.

Conflict

Suitable for: older children and adolescents

A conflict situation applying to adolescents is provided to help to teach them how to approach conflict in constructive ways. This may open up discussion about similar situations the client has become involved in, and allows the therapist to coach them through a hypothetical situation using the assertiveness skills mentioned above.

Mapping the Conflict

Suitable for: older children and adolescents

This sheet shows how to look at a conflict from many sides to determine the needs, fears and wants of all involved parties. This teaches children and adolescents to take a broad perspective on conflict and to consider the stance of others involved. This can be very effective for creating empathy and understanding towards others and for fostering an attitude of compromise.

Mediation made Simple

Suitable for: older children and adolescents

This tip sheet guides the client through the steps of mediation, providing advice on how to help the involved parties arive at a mutually agreeable solution. This is a very important skill for older children and adolescents to learn in order to navigate the complex world of social relationships they will encounter throughout their lives.

Fight–Flight

This questionnaire is designed to help you to understand your approach to communication with others, particularly in conflict situations.

Answer these questions as honestly as possible. You will act differently with different people and in different situations; however, try to think about what you do *most of the time* when you have a problem with someone.

When you have a problem with someone, do you: (*circle*)	Rarely	Sometimes	Often	Always
explode violently	0	1	2	3
call them names	0	1	2	3
shout	0	1	2	3
interrupt them	0	1	2	3
insist you are right	0	1	2	3
talk over the other person	0	1	2	3
prove your point	0	1	2	3
argue	0	1	2	3
criticise them	0	1	2	3
threaten the other to 'do it or else'	0	1	2	3
get even	0	1	2	3
Add up your score – FIGHT TOTAL				

Fight–Flight *cont.*

Now try these questions:

When you have a problem with someone, do you: (*circle*)	Rarely	Sometimes	Often	Always
take it out on someone else	0	1	2	3
talk about them behind their back	0	1	2	3
pretend nothing is wrong	0	1	2	3
give them the 'silent treatment'	0	1	2	3
tell yourself you shouldn't be upset	0	1	2	3
dwell on how mean/bad/awful they are	0	1	2	3
withdraw from them or avoid them	0	1	2	3
get sad and upset	0	1	2	3
pretend it doesn't matter	0	1	2	3
hope the problem goes away	0	1	2	3
try to be extra nice to that person	0	1	2	3
Add up your score – FLIGHT TOTAL				

Which were you highest on – **Fight** or **Flight?** _____

- If you were highest on **fight**, you have a **confrontational** approach to conflict. This means that you probably get very angry and attacking towards others, you like to be right and you want to win at all costs.

- If you were higher on **flight**, you have an **avoidant** approach to conflict. This means that you find conflict very uncomfortable and will do anything to prevent it. You will let the other win just to keep the peace.

Assertiveness

To be assertive, you just need to speak up for yourself in a way that does not disrespect the other person. You neither fight nor run away – you FLOW!

For those who prefer FLIGHT: It is hard for some people to speak up for themselves but it is very important. So if someone has done something that makes you feel uncomfortable, you owe it to yourself to speak up rather than ignoring it. Start speaking up about little things and gradually build up to more difficult things.

For those who FIGHT: You need to tone down your approach and only speak from your perspective and feelings. Remember to always respect the other and to keep in mind that you want to keep this relationship in the future.

Assertiveness tips – how to flow

- Go away and think about what is upsetting you before you approach the other person.

- Write down what you want to say first and practise it on someone else to get their feedback.

- Use an 'I' statement to make sure you express yourself clearly and from your own perspective:

    I feel _____ (your emotion)

    When you _____ (what they do that upsets you)

    I would like _____ (what you want them to do differently)

Assertiveness *cont.*

- Ask the other person if you can talk to them.

- Talk to them ALONE – don't include others.

- Remember that above all else, you want to keep this friendship and that most people wouldn't hurt your feelings on purpose.

- Remember that if something upsets you, you have a right to speak up about it – don't chicken out!

- Keep your voice calm and low.

- Stick to your point.

- Look the other person in the eye.

- Stand up straight so that you look confident – even if you don't feel it!

- Give them the benefit of the doubt – they may not have done anything on purpose, so your comments may come as a surprise.

- If they don't seem to be hearing you, repeat your message calmly and clearly and then let it go.

- Sometimes, people need to go away and think about it before they can fully understand your point.

Saying 'NO'

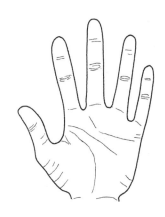

Saying 'NO' to a friend can be really hard, especially if you think they will be angry with you. If a friend of yours wants you to do something that you don't want to do, you need to be prepared to stand up for what you know is right.

This can be hard but you mustn't do anything you don't feel comfortable with, so here are some ways to say 'NO' if you need to:

Ways to say 'NO'	Reasons to give for saying 'NO'
• 'No thanks!' • 'No way!' • 'Count me out this time.' • 'No, but instead, what if we do…?' • 'I don't THINK so!' • 'What?! Are you crazy??' • 'No, not for me.' • 'No thanks, I'm not into that.' • 'I don't want to be mean.' • 'I'm not like that.'	• 'I'm already in trouble.' • 'It's not worth the risk.' • 'I like being with you, but I don't want to do this.' • 'No, I'd rather…' • 'My parents would kill me!' • 'I'm trying to be good!' • 'I don't want to get caught.' • 'If we got caught I wouldn't be able to do…' • 'It's really upsetting him/her.'

Saying 'NO' *cont.*

Imagine yourself in these situations. How could you say 'NO'?

1. Some of your friends are going to skip maths class by saying they're going to the toilet, but they plan to meet up elsewhere. They ask you to join in but you don't want to.

Your answer:

2. A friend offers you a cigarette and you don't want it.

Your answer:

Conflict

SARAH is having a birthday party but her parents have told her she can only have twenty people over. She has eight boys she wants to ask and twenty girls in her group from school. She wants to have them all but her parents have been really firm about it, and threatened to cancel the whole thing if she asked to have any more people. She narrows it down to five boys but she still has to exclude five girls. The five girls she plans to exclude are fairly new group members and Sarah is not as close to them as her other friends. However, some of these girls have heard about the party and Sarah knows they will be hurt not to be invited.

ROBERT has been a close friend of Sarah's since primary school and is invited to her party, but can't go because it's his mother's birthday dinner on the same night. He feels really bad because he wants to go to both, but knows he has to be at his mum's dinner. Sarah is really mad at him for saying he can't go to her party. Sarah is not talking to him so he feels annoyed at her and tries to avoid her by hanging out with other friends.

CLAIRE has just joined Sarah's group this term and hasn't been invited to the party. She supposes it is because Sarah doesn't know her very well but it still hurts to be left out. She feels really alone but doesn't want to ask if she can go because she feels rejected. It is hard when the party is all anyone talks about anymore.

TINA is also invited to Sarah's party but the boy she likes is not. She feels annoyed about this. Tina is also friends with Claire and the other four girls who have not been invited out of their group. She feels stuck in the middle because she can't talk about the party in front of the girls who haven't been invited and she's not sure if she even wants to go anymore. She is stuck in between Sarah and the girls who have been left out and is feeling a lot of tension.

What is the shared problem here?

List each person's needs and fears on the 'Mapping the Conflict' sheet.

Can you find a solution?

Mapping the Conflict

Who: _____

Needs: _____

_____

_____

Fears: _____

_____

_____

Wants: _____

Who: _____

Needs: _____

_____

_____

Fears: _____

_____

_____

Wants: _____

THE PROBLEM

_____

_____

_____

_____

_____

_____

_____

_____

Who: _____

Needs: _____

_____

_____

Fears: _____

_____

_____

Wants: _____

Who: _____

Needs: _____

_____

_____

Fears: _____

_____

_____

Wants: _____

Mediation made Simple

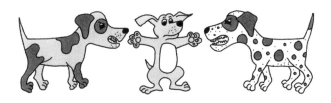

Follow these steps to role-play how James could help mediate between his friends to resolve their conflict. As the mediator, James needs to:

1. Set rules

a. Explain that he is on no-one's side and that no-one is right or wrong, that all people are entitled to their feelings.

b. Make it clear that a solution must be found to the problem so that they can all move on.

c. Stress that they will have to be willing to compromise to reach a solution.

d. Set clear rules about no interrupting, name-calling, or blaming. People are to speak one at a time and to listen to each other.

2. Listen to everyone

a. Explain that everyone's opinion is valid and deserves to be heard.

b. Each person is to express their needs, fears, and what they want, one at a time.

c. Make sure that all listen and do not interrupt, argue or judge.

d. Encourage each person to repeat what is said (paraphrasing) to make sure they understand the speaker.

3. Resolve the conflict

a. The mediator then guides each person to make a suggestion to resolve the conflict.

b. Remind all people that compromise and understanding are important in resolving conflict.

c. Help an agreement to be reached.

d. All must commit to the agreement.

6.3 Safety and empowerment

In this section, ideas are given for dealing with relational aggression and bullying in peer relationships. Bullying is an issue that can cause children and adolescents enormous stress and can significantly affect their interpersonal relationships and their self-concept. For these reasons, the skills in this section aim to educate children about bullying and to empower them to deal with it in an assertive manner.

Bullying Behaviours

Suitable for: any age

This sheet starts by defining bullying and then provides room for the child or adolescent client to generate ideas about bullying behaviours in four categories: physical, verbal, social and psychological. This sheet aims to highlight the many forms of bullying and relational aggression so that young people can be aware of their own and others' actions and identify bullying early.

Power

Suitable for: older children and adolescents

This exercise asks the child to think about what makes one person more powerful than another. This can open up discussion about peer dynamics, family systems and self-esteem, and can allow the therapist to gain insight into the client's interpersonal relationships and their beliefs about their own personal power.

Bullying Survival Guide

Suitable for: older children and adolescents

This guide contains many tips and hints for dealing with bullying situations. Three options are given for coping with intimidating behaviour by peers. To be most effective, the appropriate response could be discussed with the therapist and role-played in session. It is also important that the therapist discusses other options for remaining safe at school and at home, so that the client has many options for preserving their safety and security.

Bullying Scenarios

Suitable for: older children and adolescents

Three typical relational aggression scenarios are provided for use in role-plays or as a springboard for discussion about coping strategies.

Stopping Aggression in Friendships

Suitable for: older children and adolescents

Aggression within friendships is a common issue affecting children and adolescents. It is especially difficult to deal with because it is not recognised as bullying (and often isn't), but it can still create power and control dynamics and cause unhappiness. This sheet guides the child client through an approach to relational aggression using an assertive 'I' statement.

Bystanders

Suitable for: older children and adolescents

This sheet emphasises the role of bystanders in supporting bullying behaviour. It explains why this supports bullying and how to make a stand to prevent bullying.

Safety Plan

Suitable for: any age

This plan could be completed by the child with the therapist in order to clarify behaviours which are not considered safe for the child and what actions they should take should they find themselves in an unsafe situation. This is very important for children in domestic violence or abuse situations who need to know what is OK and what is not, and exactly what to do if they are in danger.

Safe People, Safe Feelings

Suitable for: any age

This sheet draws young children's attention to their personal feelings of safety. It asks them to list the people who make them feel safe and the people who make them feel unsafe. It is important for the therapist to listen carefully to the child's responses and to validate their feelings should they describe a person in their life. The therapist can encourage the child to observe and trust their subjective feelings of anxiety and to take steps to keep themselves safe should they need to.

Many children are not aware of their physical cues of anxiety and put themselves in situations where they trust a person who makes them feel uncomfortable. This can make them vulnerable to abuse. For children who describe a person who makes them feel threatened, this sheet, along with discussion with the therapist, can teach them that they have the right to feel safe and that they can speak up and be listened to any time they feel unsafe.

Bullying Behaviours

BULLYING: Repeated intimidation over a period of time conducted by a more powerful person towards a less powerful person. It may include physical, verbal, psychological or relational aggression. It can be conducted by an individual or a group and the recipient often feels unable to defend themselves.

Physical	Verbal
Social	**Psychological**

Power

What makes one person more powerful than another?

-
-
-
-
-
-
-
-
-

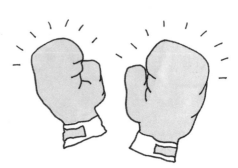

Why do these things give them power?

How could one person use their power to bully or control another?

Bullying Survival Guide

If you think people are purposely trying to make you feel uncomfortable and you think they might be bullying you, DON'T FEAR – there are several options for stopping it!

The first thing to remember is that **no-one** has the right to intimidate you.

Option 1: you decide to talk to them

- If you think you can, go up to one of them and ask if there is a problem. Calmly say to them **'I've noticed you are...(staring at me/talking about me/laughing at me)...and it makes me feel bad. I was wondering if you have a problem you want to talk about.'**

- This means that they have to explain themselves! If they are not trying to hurt you, they will probably be surprised and give an explanation. If they are trying to hurt you, they most likely will deny that they were doing anything.

- It is still worth it, though – it lets them know you will speak up and that you are not an easy target.

- This will not be the option that everyone would choose – it is HARD!

Option 2: ignore them and get help

- If you think that saying something won't work, then you need to **ignore them**. Never let them know that you are aware of what they are doing. **Never give them the thrill of knowing they have upset you**.

- Have fun with your own friends and don't focus on the bullies – don't be tempted to bully them back. They will probably get bored and find something else to interest themselves.

Bullying Survival Guide *cont.*

- **Tell someone:** a teacher you trust, a parent, a friend.

- **Don't keep it all inside and blame yourself.** You are not alone, others can and will help you – it will not make things worse.

- **Write down** (or print out) anything they say or do to you that you are uncomfortable with. This means that you have evidence and examples to back up your case.

Option 3: when you are caught off guard by them

- If you are confronted by a bully (e.g. If they say something mean to you or say something loud enough for you to hear) you need to **remain calm, don't let them know it has upset you.**

- **Turn** and face them and calmly **look** at them for **three whole seconds** – this will show that you are not scared or intimidated.

- **THEN**, in a **calm voice** with **a puzzled** facial expression, say **'You know, it is really sad that you feel the need to put me down just to feel better about yourself,'** and calmly walk away!

- This is powerful because it shows that you know what they are doing, that you don't respect their actions, and that you are not intimidated by them. **Trust me – it works!!**

Bullying Scenarios

Scenario 1

Each afternoon you travel home on the same train as a group of older kids from your school. Each time you take your seat, they move over and tell you to move and that the seat belongs to them. Each time you move, but no matter where you sit, they continue this intimidating behaviour. This goes on every afternoon for three weeks.

What do you do?

Scenario 2

At a recent school dance you talk to a girl that your best friend likes. Feeling threatened, he warns you away from her and lets you know that he will not be your friend if you talk to her again. On the following Monday, you return to school to find that everyone in your group has been told that you have stolen this girl from your friend and you were seen with her outside the dance. Apparently, your friend emailed this to twenty of your friends. They are all furious with you. A week later, he sends them all another set of lies about you and this girl. No-one believes you when you say it's not true.

What do you do?

Scenario 3

You and three friends all audition for parts in the school musical. You are selected and they are not. Suddenly, your friends start to distance themselves from you. In the school yard, they turn away when you come over to say hi, whisper to each other when you are nearby and give you death stares whenever you mention the musical. They have a party and invite the whole group except you, and gradually, you notice other girls pulling away from you as well.

What do you do?

Stopping Aggression in Friendships

No friendship is perfect, BUT friendships are *not* supposed to make you feel bad about yourself, to make you cry, or to feel constantly under pressure to be a certain way or to do certain things. If this is happening in any of your friendships you need to SPEAK UP and put a stop to it!

To do this you need to:

- remember you deserve to be treated fairly in your friendships

- remember that no-one should make you feel bad in a friendship

- remember that friendships should give you more good feelings than bad

- remember that it is OK to have lots of friends

- remember that you don't need to have just one 'best friend'

- stand up for yourself and act confidently!

- hold your head up high

- look the other firmly in the eye

- stand up tall and straight

- not look intimidated

- tell them what is bothering you in a fair and respectful way – use an **'I' Message!**

'I' Messages

I feel _____ (your emotion)

When you _____ (what they do that upsets you)

I would like _____ (what you want them to do differently)

Try these examples:

1. Caitlin feels pressured by Britt to exclude Kate. What could she say to Britt?

I feel _____

When you _____

I would like _____

2. Sam was the only one not invited to Andrew's party. What could he say to Andrew?

I felt _____

When you _____

I would like _____

Now try your own 'I' Message for a situation where a friend has upset you.

I feel _____

When you _____

I would like _____

Bystanders

What to do to stop bullying

Bullying is not just a problem between the bully and the victim – it is a problem that most often happens **in front of others**. People who witness bullying may feel uncomfortable but not know what to do. They may be drawn into it and end up bullying themselves. People who are 'just watching' may be letting the bully think that they **approve** when they don't.

Most instances of bullying involve bystanders, but very few of these people do anything about it. Most people feel uncomfortable witnessing bullying, but very few are ever brave enough to try to stop it.

Bullies thrive on an audience. They feel powerful and impressive when others watch their display of dominance. It is their way of saying 'See how powerful and cool I am? Don't get on the wrong side of me or I could do this to you!'

Don't let them have this chance, **be brave and stand up for the victim**. If you say or do nothing, you are approving of what is happening. No-one likes to be bullied, remember this when you see it happening to someone else and **DO SOMETHING!!**

If **everyone** took a stand, bullies would be out-numbered – you have the power to put an end to bullying, especially if all bystanders **took a stand together!**

Try these ideas:

- Don't laugh – this shows approval for the bully.

- Don't watch – walk away from the bullying. If the bully has no audience, they will not get any satisfaction from bullying.

- Go and tell a staff member/parent that someone is being bullied.

- If the bully is a friend of yours, try saying:

    'Leave her / him alone.'
    'That's too far.'
    'Let it go.'
    'Don't be mean.'

- If the bully is not a friend of yours, try saying:

    'You are only making yourself look bad by doing that to him / her.'
    'Are you getting satisfaction out of that?'
    'Being mean won't get you any friends, you know.'

- Above all else **DON'T JOIN IN** at any cost. Remember what it feels like to be the victim of bullying. **IT HURTS** – so don't become a bully yourself and don't encourage bullies by watching them at work.

Safety Plan

Safe behaviours:

Unsafe behaviours:

What to do when I feel unsafe:

Safe people

_____ Phone: _____

_____ Phone: _____

_____ Phone: _____

Safe People, Safe Feelings

List the names of some people who you feel safe with:

Why do they make you feel safe?

How would you know if a person was unsafe?

What would they do to you to make you feel unsafe?

How do you feel in your body when you are around them?

What could you do if you felt unsafe around someone?

DESSERT

SECTION 7 FAMILY ISSUES

7.1 Family story

Families are complex emotional melting-pots that can provide enormous support and encouragement or provoke enormous upheaval and distress. In order to improve cohesion in the family, it is vital for the therapist to gain a clear picture of the family's history, each family member's role, and the general patterns of communication and power within the family. The process of telling the family 'story' can be therapeutic in itself, as it allows for reflection and appreciation of the strength of the family and each of its members. The strategies in this section could be used with any kind of family unit (nuclear, step, blended or split) to explore their history and their presenting issues.

Family of Origin

Suitable for: any age

This exercise is designed for the parents or parental figures to complete and then to discuss with the rest of the family. It aims to encourage each parent to reflect upon their experiences in their family of origin and the lessons they learned about themselves and about parenting. This then allows them to think about the relevance of their early lessons for their current family. For instance, a parent who learned to 'be seen and not heard' while they were growing up might unwittingly expect total obedience in their children now. Upon reflection, they might realise that this is an unrealistic expectation and that it is causing significant distress within their family.

It is the role of the therapist to validate each parent's early experience of parenting and to form links where possible between that experience and the current difficulties in the family, but to do this in a non-judgemental manner. By acknowledging and validating each parent's experience, the therapist models for the rest of the family how to be accepting and understanding of other family members' past experiences. This activity aims to create an atmosphere of understanding and insight in order to diffuse blame and anger and to focus the family on productivity and change.

Our Family Story

Suitable for: any age

This activity asks the family to depict their family story in the form of a genogram (family tree). This requires the use of symbols, colours, lines and captions to depict relationships throughout the history of their family as far back as they can remember.

Telling the family story through a genogram can be an extremely valuable tool for creating connectedness and understanding within the family. The sheet provided explains how to draw a genogram, but the therapist will need to provide a large sheet of paper and coloured pens to allow the family the space to do this exercise justice.

This activity gives the therapist a wealth of information about the family's history and about the way the family executes a task together. It is helpful for the family to explain their story to the therapist as they record it onto the genogram, and for the therapist to validate the experiences of the family as a unit by drawing on strengths.

Draw your Family

Suitable for: any age

This activity is a simplified version of the genogram. The family is asked to draw the family unit, depicting each member as a symbol. This focuses mainly on the immediate family but other significant people (such as grandparents) could be depicted as well. This activity provides an opportunity for the therapist to observe the family working on a task together, as well as gaining valuable information about each family member as perceived by others.

Roles within the Family

Suitable for: any age

This sheet allows the therapist to explore the roles within the family by asking what role each family member plays in the family. It might be interesting to note any disparity between how one member sees their role and how the rest of the family sees their role. Communication patterns will become evident during the exercise, giving the therapist more information about power dynamics within the family.

Strengths of each Family Member

Suitable for: any age

In this exercise the family is encouraged to think about the strengths of each individual family member. As an assessment tool, this exercise provides much information about the family's ability to acknowledge strengths, to praise its members, and to negotiate within its ranks. If the family works cooperatively, it will be a very positive exercise. If the family finds this task difficult this could indicate an area to work on in therapy. Either way, it gives the therapist a clear baseline of the family's functioning and level of support for one another.

Family of Origin

Describe your family when you were a child. Who was there? How did your family members relate to each other? What parenting style did your parents use?

What did you learn about parenting from your father/father figure?

What did you learn about parenting from your mother/mother figure?

Which of these lessons are still relevant for your family today?

Our Family Story

Most families have complicated and interesting pasts. Draw your family tree to illustrate your family history!

1. Start with your current family unit. Draw in each family member, using these symbols:

For males: □   For females: ○   Deceased: ⊠ ⊗

Married

Children:

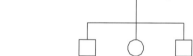

Divorced:
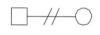

Separated:
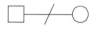

Remarried:
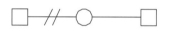

Conflict:

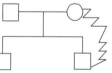

Strong relationship:

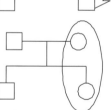

2. Then move on to each parent's siblings and their families, using the same symbols.

3. Finally, draw in the grandparents and their siblings (if you can remember them).

Draw your Family

In the space below, draw your family. Think of a symbol to represent each person. Include all the members of the family that are important to the family as a whole.

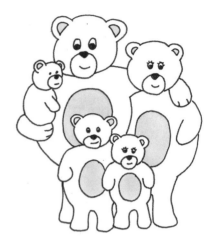

Roles within the Family

Put each family member's name in the left column and what their role in the family is in the right column.

Family member	Role in the family

Strengths of each Family Member

Put each family member's name in the left column and write some of their good qualities and strengths in the right column.

Family member	Strengths

7.2 Connectedness

Helping families to reconnect is an important and rewarding part of family therapy. The exercises and activities in this section aim to encourage families to interact in a positive manner, to enjoy one another's company and to foster an atmosphere of trust and support within the family.

All Aboard!

Suitable for: any age

This activity illustrates how connected a family is when given a difficult situation to deal with. It does this by forcing the family to occupy an ever diminishing physical space (outlined by a rope on the ground), thus compelling them to support each other in order to achieve the goal. The therapist's role is to make an area on the floor no bigger than one metre square and to ask the whole family to fit themselves into this space. The therapist observes how the family does this, then asks them to step out of the rope area and reduces the size of the space before asking the family to fit themselves into it again. This continues until the therapist feels that the family has had to work together to support each other in order to occupy a very small space.

It is then the role of the therapist to debrief the exercise by encouraging the family members to reflect upon the manner in which they worked together, supported each other and communicated with each other in order to complete the task. The sheet contains some reflective questions to guide this process. This activity is a useful assessment tool for therapists, as well as a therapeutic and fun exercise for families.

What we Love and Appreciate about...

Suitable for: any age

In this activity, each family member is given one of these sheets and writes their name on it. Each sheet then gets passed around the family, with each family member writing something that they love and appreciate about that person on it.

When the sheets are returned to their owners, they will have a compliment from each family member on them. These compliments are then read out for the whole family to hear. This activity can be very powerful in connecting and validating each family member.

The therapist can ensure the success of this task by choosing the right time to execute it (not in a time of crisis or extreme hostility!) and by setting some groundrules. Some helpful groundrules are: be honest with your compliments, be specific, don't add 'but' onto the end of compliments, and think deeply about what you appreciate about the other. At the completion of the sharing of compliments, it can be helpful to go around the group, asking each family member how it felt for them to receive their compliments and what they meant to them.

Fun Activities for Families

Suitable for: any age

This sheet gives some examples of fun activities that families could do together to increase their connection. It then asks the family to think up for themselves a long list of fun activities that they could do. It is important that all family members are involved in this discussion and that all ideas are validated, rather than discounted as too expensive or silly. Finally, the sheet asks them to think about why these activities might be good for their family.

Family Members' Needs

Suitable for: any age

In this exercise, the concept of individual needs is raised. It would be helpful for the therapist to guide initial discussion about needs and to explain that each person in the family has certain things that they need in order to feel happy in their life. Then the therapist addresses each family member and asks them what they need to feel happy in their life. This could be things that they need from the family, such as freedom, understanding and respect, as well as things they need from outside the family, such as balance between school or work and socialising. The therapist can be the scribe who records each person's needs on the sheet.

The purpose of this exercise is to create honest sharing of needs in an atmosphere of understanding and collaboration. This can lead to problem-solving and goal-setting in order to meet as many of the family members' needs as possible. In addition, this activity creates empathy and understanding among family members and precludes typecasting them into particular roles.

All Aboard!

How did you feel about having to squeeze into a small space with your family?

How well do you think the family worked together to achieve the goal of fitting into a small area?

How good was your family's communication during this task?

Do you think the family was supportive of all the family members?

Did anyone take on specific roles during this activity?

Do you think your family needs to improve its connection? How?

What we Love and Appreciate about...

Write something that you love and appreciate about _____ on this sheet:

Fun Activities for Families

Having fun together is really important for having a healthy family. Here are some suggestions for fun activities that you could do all together:

- **outings:** picnics, park, zoo, shopping, cafés, ice-cream

- **day trips:** bushwalking, driving, beach, country

- **holidays:** camping, weekends away

- **at home:** videos, games, sports, art and craft, cooking, walking the dog, washing the car, talking, gardening.

Can you think of any fun activities that your family could do?

Why would these activities be good for your family?

Family Members' Needs

Family member	Needs from life e.g. *balance between work and home life*	Needs from family e.g. *understanding and respect*

7.3 Parenting

This section contains information to assist the therapist in some important components of parent-training. The skills described here all aim to increase assertiveness and cohesion within the family, thereby reducing the frequency and severity of conflict and aggression. For any parenting strategy to be effective, it needs to be clearly explained to the child, consistently applied by all parental figures as a united front, and backed up with appropriate rewards and consequences.

Praise

Suitable for: any age

This sheet prompts the parent (with or without help from the child) to think of all the behaviours they could praise in their child. This list should include behaviours the child already does, as well as behaviours the parent would like to see more of. It is important that the therapist shape the parent's responses to ensure that they are specific, behaviour-based and realistic. Second, this exercise asks the parent and the child to list all the ways the parent could praise the child. This is to include verbal responses such as 'Good job!', nonverbal responses such as a smile or attention, and material rewards such as chocolate or small prizes!

The aim of this activity is for the parent to be specific about what to praise and how to praise, and for the child to know exactly what it is their parent expects from them, and what signals their parent will use to show approval. This makes it much easier for the child to do the right thing and for their parent to respond appropriately, thus improving their relationship and increasing the child's self-esteem.

Setting Limits

Suitable for: any age

This sheet explains why setting limits (rules) is important for parents of children and teenagers. It also explains how to set limits in place and how to back those limits up with appropriate consequences. This allows for discussion about the importance of having clear expectations and making those explicit to children. Many parents are not clear about what they expect or about the consequences of rule-breaking with their children. This results in confusion and inconsistency for the children and a lack of legitimacy and believability in parenting.

House Rules

Suitable for: any age

This sheet provides a framework for setting house rules that apply to all family members. This is important for improving the consistency of parenting and the clarity of expectations within the family home. This exercise makes parents think about how they would like the home to run and the standards of behaviour expected of all family members. With this in mind, it is advantageous if all the rules can apply to all family members. An example of a good house rule is:

Treat each other with respect – no swearing, name calling or aggression. Speak calmly, ask if you want to borrow something, look after other people's possessions.

This rule is stated in global terms and it is also specific about the behaviours that are appropriate and inappropriate, and so all family members know which behaviours are acceptable and unacceptable. Parents might also need to put in place some consequences for rule-breaking and some rewards for compliance. Not all rules will need tangible rewards because they may be general expectations of family life (and as such can be rewarded with verbal praise), but this can be guided by the parents and the therapist.

Communicating with Teenagers

Suitable for: adolescents

This tip sheet briefly describes the developmental tasks of adolescence and why communication with adolescents can be so difficult for parents. It aims to educate parents about some of the reasons behind adolescent–parent conflict and to alter parents' view of their teen. By increasing parents' understanding of the issues facing their teen, this exercise aims to reduce their reactivity towards them and therefore to reduce the frequency of conflict in the home.

Improving Communication with Teenagers

Suitable for: adolescents

This sheet lists some strategies for improving communication with young people. These suggestions might serve to prevent or better manage parent–adolescent conflict and encourage a more cohesive and mutually respectful home environment.

Family Discussion Time

Suitable for: any age

This sheet explains the concept of having a family discussion time where families can sit down together and assertively discuss issues affecting them either individually or as a family. This is an important skill for families to learn in order to be able to raise and resolve issues in a productive way. This time is also important for increasing the connection between family members through hearing about people's week and catching up, planning family outings and fun time, or making important decisions that affect the family as a whole. The sheet explains some of the guidelines that need to be adhered to by all family members in order for family discussion time to be productive. It might be useful for the therapist to explain this skill and to practise the principles in session to be sure that all family members understand.

Divorce and Separation 1

Suitable for: any age

This tip sheet contains information for parents about how children react to tension and change in the family home, and how to tell children and young people that you are separating or divorcing. This is important for pre-empting any emotional issues that might arise in these difficult circumstances.

Divorce and Separation 2

Suitable for: any age

This second sheet on divorce and separation provides advice for the parent who leaves the family home and for parents who have new partners. This might help to reduce some of the discomfort and distress caused to children when one of their parents leaves the home or begins a new relationship.

✓

Praise

We all like to receive praise for a job well done. Praise increases the likelihood of that behaviour happening again. With this in mind, answer the two following questions:

What behaviours could you praise your child for?

What are some of the different ways you could praise your child?

Setting Limits

As a parent, it can be very difficult saying NO to your child, especially if it leads to tantrums, fights and tension. Despite this, setting limits is very important for being in control, feeling respected, and for your accountability as a parent.

Here are some suggestions for setting clear limits.

- Be VERY clear about what you expect of your child's behaviour, spell this out for them. Do not expect them to guess!

- Be VERY clear about what will happen if the rules you have set in place are broken.

- Make these consequences short, sharp and meaningful to the child. For instance, when a rule is broken, you need to follow through immediately with the consequence that you threatened, and that consequence needs to be sufficiently significant for the child to deter them from doing the forbidden behaviour again.

- Never threaten without following through! This teaches your child not to respect the limits you set in place.

- Only set a limit that you mean – be prepared to follow through. For instance, if you say 'Stop fighting or we will go home', be prepared to go home immediately if the fighting does not stop!

- Plan ahead for trouble spots and set clear rules in place beforehand. For example, if long car trips always result in fighting between your children set a rule of 'No yelling, hitting or rudeness' before you leave and put a consequence in place for any rule-breaking.

- Be sure to reward rule-following to increase this as well.

Setting Limits *cont.*

What limits do you need to set for your children?

For each rule, pick a consequence that will be meaningful but that you can act upon if needed:

House Rules

Think of four or five general family rules that could apply to all family members in your house.

Be sure to describe what is acceptable and unacceptable in terms of behaviours e.g. *Treat each other with respect – no swearing, name calling or aggression. Speak calmly, ask if you want to borrow something, look after other people's possessions.*

House rule	Consequence for rule-breaking	Reward for rule following

Communicating with Teenagers

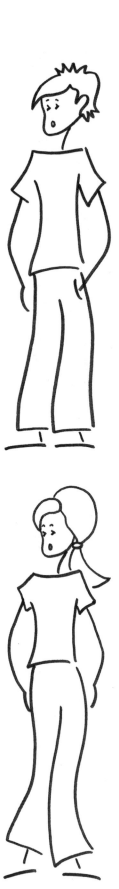

Developmental tasks of adolescence

Adolescents are going through a very difficult stage of their life, where subconsciously they are trying to create distance between themselves and their parents in order to develop into an independent adult. However, they do not have the emotional awareness or communication skills to be able to understand or express their needs in a calm and assertive manner. This means that they show their need for distance from the family through their behaviour!

Striving for independence and autonomy

When teens start to withdraw from the family and make requests for more freedom, they are trying to establish their independence. They begin to place all their attention onto their friends and start to look to their friends for confirmation that they are OK as a person (a role previously held by the family). Therefore, pleasing their friends becomes very important. This is often the cause of many arguments because teens want to push the limits set by their parents in order to please their friends.

Parents' reactions

Many parents feel that their teenager's focus on their friends and their withdrawal from the family is a personal rejection. This leads to hurt feelings and misunderstandings. Often parents feel very much taken for granted during this time, which can lead to resentment. Teenagers are in a very self-centred phase of their development where they need to gain independence from the family, and this can be interpreted as a sign that they no longer care about their family. It is important to remember that this is not the case.

Moodiness and self-esteem

When adolescents become sullen and grumpy, this is often as a result of their own self-doubt and from feeling 'not good enough'. If parents react with anger, the young person's belief about themselves is confirmed. It is important for parents to try not to take normal adolescent 'grumpiness' and withdrawal from the family as a personal rejection, but rather to see it as a crucial phase in the teenager's development into an adult.

Improving Communication with Teenagers

Here are some tips to improve your communication with your teenaged child.

- Try to think back to your own experience of adolescence and what you found difficult at that time.

- Remember that they are facing one of the most difficult times of their life, so give them a little leeway if they are grumpy or moody.

- Expect a certain standard of respectful behaviour – do not tolerate rudeness or inconsiderateness but allow them space to be alone.

- Have clear expectations of them, don't expect them to just 'know' what you want them to do.

- Be prepared to compromise on some rules. This will give your teen a feeling of control and democracy, thereby making them more likely to stick to the rules.

- Remember that while it might not be apparent, your approval is still very important to them, so be positive about their good qualities, acknowledge their strengths, and praise their efforts.

- Start to let them solve their own problems, support them but don't try to have all the answers.

- Be ready to give them your time and attention on the rare occasions that they request it! Create opportunities for them to talk.

- Don't take things too seriously; laugh and joke with your teen!

- Try not to criticise their friends, this is a sure-fire way to get off-side with your teen.

- Increase their amount of freedom in return for an increase in their amount of responsibility.

- Remember how fragile their self-esteem is at this time and never criticise them as a person or for their physical appearance.

- You don't have to love their behaviour, but they need you to love them as a person regardless. This will help them to form a healthy self-esteem.

Family Discussion Time

It is important that a family discusses issues and concerns in a calm and productive way. Setting aside some time on a regular basis to do this can promote sharing of problems, which can prevent a build-up of tension in the family.

This time doesn't have to be used to just discuss problems. It can be used to catch up, to talk about each person's week, to plan family outings and fun time, or to make decisions that affect the whole family (such as the next holiday, colours to paint the house, whether to get a dog, etc.).

To do this well, there must be guidelines that all family members agree to follow:

- All family members must participate. If one family member does not have an issue to raise, they must still be present and listen to the others.

- One person at a time shares and all others listen.

- No interrupting.

- Express concerns in a calm manner. Speak from your own perspective with no blaming, accusing or aggression.

- All must work together to find solutions to issues.

The family discussion should ideally not be longer than half-an-hour. Any issues that can't be resolved might need to be left and brought up at another time in order to resolve them. Try to incorporate a fun activity into your family discussion and include positive topics as well, so that family members do not see the discussion as an uncomfortable, unpleasant task.

Family Discussion Time *cont.*

To plan your next family discussion:

When would you have it?

Where?

What issues would you want to raise?

Divorce and Separation 1

Children's and young people's reaction to change

When there is tension and change within the family home, children often become unsettled and anxious. Different children will express this in different ways. Some children will clearly show their anxiety through clingy behaviour and through the development of a range of worries and concerns that demand your attention.

Other children will keep their fears inside and privately worry, while pretending on the outside that everything is fine. The toll can be great upon these children without anyone knowing they are suffering. Some young people withdraw and become sullen. This may be interpreted as anger by some parents.

Another group of children react to this change by demanding attention by any means necessary. This can be anything from getting into trouble, to picking fights with siblings, or through risk-taking and reckless behaviour.

Telling your child that you are separating/divorcing

However your children react to tension and change in the family home, all children will notice it and will need some explanation. If possible, it is best if both parents can tell the children together that they are going to separate or divorce. This needs to be done earlier rather than later, because children and young people are very good at picking up on what is happening and should not be left guessing. This will only create more distress, no matter how much parents try to keep the family environment 'normal'.

Often, the children will be aware that there is an issue but might not have allowed themselves to become upset about it until they are told. Even for children and young people who knew separation was coming, it is still upsetting for them. This means that parents need to give children and young people time and space to react in whatever way is best for them at the time.

The most important message your children need to hear is that both parents love them and will continue being their parents, even if you no longer all live together.

Their immediate concern after that will be where everyone will live. They will need to be reassured about staying in contact with the parent they will no longer be living with full-time and both parents need to have a clear plan about this to be ready to answer these questions.

Divorce and Separation 2

Parent relationship

When parents decide to separate or divorce, it is stressful for the children. The children's priority is usually on maintaining a good relationship with both parents regardless of where everyone decides to live.

Therefore, as parents it is absolutely VITAL that neither of you says anything negative about the other (no matter how subtle you think you are being) in front of the children or young people. They need to be allowed to love each parent in order to emerge from this situation in the healthiest way possible.

Parents must allow the children to be sad or unhappy if they need to be. Tell them that this is OK and that you will always be there for them. If they are allowed to have a healthy reaction to the loss and change, they are more likely to recover quickly. Children should not feel that they have to stifle their reaction for fear of upsetting one parent.

For the parent who moves out of the family home

Make sure that the children know that they have a place in your new home. Show them where their room is and allow them to bring whatever possessions they need to make themselves feel at home. Explain that the rules at your house might be a bit different from those they are used to. Be very clear about those rules and expectations, because the change from one home to another can be hard enough for children, without having an unspoken set of new and different rules to contend with.

It can be helpful to have special toys or possessions at the new house to make them feel at home, and extras of essentials (such as certain items of clothing and toiletries) so that they do not feel that they are 'living out of a suitcase' at the new house.

Parents with new partners

The most important thing that children need to know is that your new partner does not in any way threaten the relationship they have with you. Make spending time alone with your children a priority if you do have a new partner, to show them that you are still their parent first. New partners need to accommodate this in order to forge a positive relationship with each child.

7.4 Problem-solving

This section contains activities and worksheets for families to complete that encourage them to work as a team, to solve shared problems and to set collaborative goals. The aim of this section is to increase collaborative sharing of ideas within the family and appreciation of each person's contribution to problem-solving as a family.

Teamwork

Suitable for: any age

For this activity the family is asked to work together to guide one blindfolded family member from one side of the room to the other, using only verbal commands. The instructions for this exercise are outlined on the sheet but the therapist will need to provide a blindfold and any other objects that could be used to create a 'minefield' for the blindfolded client. The therapist will need to specify where the start and finish line is for the task.

This is an excellent assessment tool to allow the therapist to witness firsthand how the family approaches problems and works on tasks together. It can be helpful to leave the family alone to execute these tasks (video record the session or watch through a one-way mirror), or to observe from a discreet distance while providing no guidance.

After each family member has been guided across the room, the therapist can debrief the exercise by asking the family about what they noticed, who performed which roles, how well they felt that they worked together, and where they felt they could have improved. Following this, the therapist can also give feedback about the task: any observations they made about family members' roles and cohesion and collaboration. This is where it can be useful to have videotaped the exercise so that family members can watch themselves and see how they worked together (or not, in some cases). This can greatly aid the therapist in giving feedback.

Problem-solving

Suitable for: any age

For this exercise, the therapist might need to enlarge the problem-solving sheet onto A3-sized paper to allow for extra room. This sheet works by first looking at the 'problem' as it is for the whole family in the smallest box. For this, the therapist needs to ensure that the problem is stated in global terms and that it is not blaming or involving only one family member (e.g. 'James is rude and inconsiderate' could be reframed as 'Family fights over small things'). Next, each family member shares and records the effect of that problem on them or their issue, in relation to the problem in the second largest box. Finally, as a family, all members work together to find solutions to each person's individual issue in relation to the problem in the largest box.

This activity encourages family members to see each person's experience of the problem and to work together to find solutions to each problem. In doing so, they solve the bigger problem for the family and validate each family member in the process.

Strengths, Weaknesses, Opportunities, Threats

Suitable for: any age

This sheet asks the family to think (with the therapist's help) about their strengths and weaknesses as a family, and their opportunities for happiness and the things that threaten their happiness as a family. This promotes reflection and teamwork and allows the development of a family identity. This can be a useful revision and relapse-prevention exercise.

Goal-setting as a Family

Suitable for: any age

This table encourages families to think about what they would like to achieve over the next year and to plan those goals collaboratively. These goals could be planned and discussed at 'Family Discussion Time' (see page 215) and worked on as a family. This gives the family a sense of cohesion and a common purpose.

Teamwork

Minefield!

This activity will show how well you can work together as a team. One family member is to be blindfolded and guided from one corner of the room to the other by the rest of the family. Their journey will be timed. Each family member is to have a turn being blindfolded and guided by the others. How well can you all work together to achieve the fastest time?

1. Blindfold the first family member and spin them around three times. Lead them to the corner of the room furthest from the door and ask them to wait until prompted to move.

2. Move the chairs and any other objects in the room to alter the landscape.

3. Nominate one family member to be the timekeeper and to start timing from the moment the rest of the family tells the blindfolded participant to begin moving.

4. Guide the blindfolded person, using only voice commands. Any family member can give directions but the object is to guide them across the room in the shortest possible time. All family members giving directions must stay out of the way of the blindfolded person.

What worked well in this exercise?

What could be improved?

What did you notice about how your family completed this?

Were all family members involved?

What roles did certain family members take on?

Problem-solving

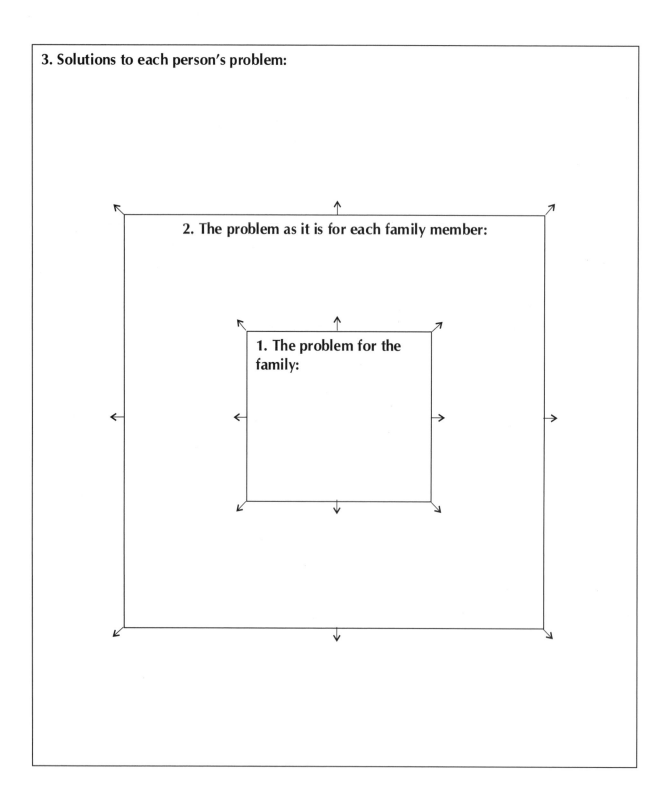

3. Solutions to each person's problem:

2. The problem as it is for each family member:

1. The problem for the family:

Strengths, Weaknesses, Opportunities, Threats

As a family, what do you see as your strengths, weaknesses, opportunities for happiness and threats to your happiness?

Strengths	Weaknesses	Opportunities	Threats

Goal-setting as a Family

As a family, what are your goals for the next year?

Goal	Why do It?	Step 1	Step 2	Step 3	Step 4

8 RESILIENCE

8.1 Building self-esteem

This is an area that can benefit most clients, but enhancing self-esteem can be a process that takes time. This section contains worksheets and activities for all age-groups to help them to begin building a more rounded sense of self-esteem. These exercises aim to provide therapists with many ideas and a variety of resources for helping their young clients to develop in this area. The activities cover a range of ages and abilities to suit most clients.

Finding my Positive Qualities

Suitable for: older children and adolescents

This sheet prompts clients to identify some of their strengths. Some clients find this extremely difficult, so the questions are geared with this in mind. It is important that the therapist affirms any disclosure and enthusiastically encourages further sharing to reinforce and encourage the client.

Good Things about ME!

Suitable for: any age

This is an unstructured sheet to allow the child or adolescent client to record their positive qualities and achievements. This allows for discussion and validation of success, no matter how great or small. This can be used as an evidence-gathering task by asking the child to interview people in their life and recording their compliments on the sheet for the child.

What Makes ME Special!

Suitable for: any age

This sheet is helpful for all age groups because it encourages clients to identify their special qualities and draw them onto the picture. It prompts the client to think about their own uniqueness and to acknowledge their positive qualities by writing them down. This can then be stuck up in a visible location to be read daily.

Nice Things People Say about ME!

Suitable for: any age

This activity asks clients to recall positive things that people in their life say about them. For the younger children, it helps them to remember all the reasons why they are praised, special and loved. For older children and adolescents, it teaches them to acknowledge compliments and to gather evidence to challenge any negative thoughts they might have about themselves. The therapist might need to write for younger children or to encourage the child to draw a symbol to describe the compliment.

Finding my Positive Qualities

What do you like about yourself?

What do you do well (not perfectly!)?

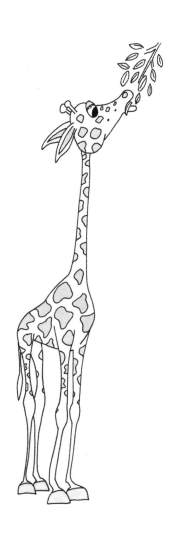

What do other people compliment you on?

What qualities do you value in others? Which do you share (even if only in some small way)?

Good Things about ME!

Write on this page all things that are good about you. Be sure to include your achievements, your good points, things you are good at and nice things that other people have said about you.

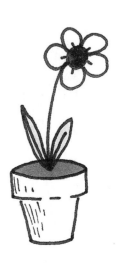

What Makes ME Special!

What are some of the things that make you special?

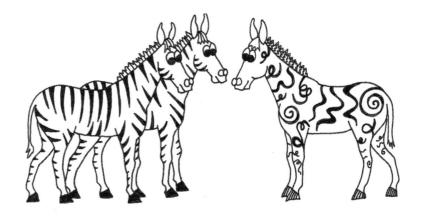

Nice Things People Say about ME!

Think about all the nice things people say about you... Write them down below!

What MUM says:

What DAD says:

What my GRANDPARENTS say:

What my TEACHER says:

What my FRIENDS say:

8.2 Body image

This section aims to address low self-esteem as a result of poor body image. Many people judge their self-worth by their outer appearance, particularly in adolescence. The sheets in this section address body-related low self-esteem by challenging the belief that the outer appearance is a measure of inner self-worth.

My Thoughts about my Body – Female

Suitable for: older children and adolescents

In this activity, the female client is asked to think about her body and to write onto the diagram the sorts of things she tells herself about specific parts of her body. This will show the therapist which areas the client criticises herself about and the language she uses when she does that.

My Thoughts about my Body – Male

Suitable for: older children and adolescents

This is the same activity for use with male clients. The client is asked to think about his body and to write onto the diagram the sorts of things he tells himself about specific parts of his body.

Pressures on Girls

Suitable for: adolescents

This activity asks female clients to think about how the 'perfect female' should look and act and where she received those messages. The aim of this exercise is to generate thought and discussion about the many influences on body image ranging from:

- the media: advertising, magazines, and television
- celebrities and role models: actors, musicians and models

- culture: stereotypes, societal expectations and gender roles
- peer influences: popularity, acceptance, dating, peer comparison and conforming to a peer group image.

With the help of the therapist, some of these influences might be challenged in order to reduce the pressure felt by the female client to look and behave in a prescribed manner.

Pressures on Guys

Suitable for: adolescents

This sheet is specifically for male clients. It explores their personal body concept and asks them to think about the increasing amount of pressure that is placed upon young men to look and act in a particular way to be 'masculine' and popular. It aims to elicit the same information as the 'Pressures on Girls' sheet, but with a specific focus on male stereotypes and expectations.

Thinking about Body Image

Suitable for: adolescents

This sheet encourages adolescents and adults (particularly females) to think about their perception of their body and the origins of the messages they hear about how they 'should' look. This could elucidate some useful information for the therapist about deeper family dynamics or the underlying belief systems behind poor body image in the female client.

Challenging Negative Body-related Thoughts

Suitable for: adolescents

This sheet guides the client through the process of challenging negative body-related thoughts by first recording self-critical thoughts, then examining the consequences of those thoughts, and finally by encouraging the client to change each thought into a more helpful, positive one.

Dispelling Diet Myths

Suitable for: adolescents

This sheet is designed to challenge some of the many diet-related myths that can lead to poor eating habits and dangerous weight loss. Supporting clients to treat their body with respect and to maintain a healthy weight is important. This sheet might help the therapist to challenge unrealistic weight loss expectations or unsafe weight loss methods. Should clients want to lose weight, they should be supported if they do this in a safe and healthy manner and for sound reasons (i.e. not to 'fit in' or to 'fix' all their problems). This sheet might encourage discussion about body image and weight issues and therefore uncover and possibly prevent harmful eating habits.

My Thoughts about my Body – Female

What do you think about your body?
What are some of the things you say to yourself about your body?
Write your thoughts onto the diagram below…

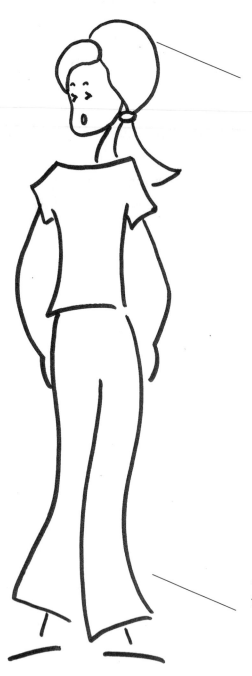

Example: When I look at my hair I think 'I hate my hair, I can't make it do anything.'

Example: I don't mind my legs, they are OK.'

My Thoughts about my Body – Male

What do you think about your body?

What are some of the things you say to yourself about your body?

Write your thoughts onto the diagram below…

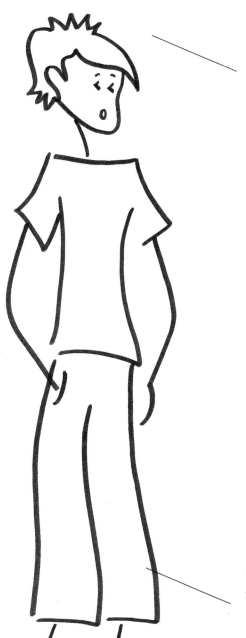

Example: When I think about my height I think 'I am too short, I wish I was taller.'

Example: I don't mind my legs, they are OK.'

Pressures on Girls

In the space below, draw the 'perfect' female.
Place captions around her describing her personality, her life and her appearance.

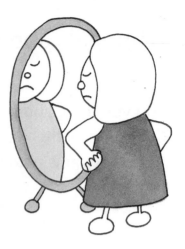

Where do you think we get this idea about how girls 'should' be? How realistic is
this?

How many people do you think actually look and act like this picture?

Do you think you should look and act like this? How does that make you feel?

Pressures on Guys

In the space below, draw the 'perfect' male. Place captions around him describing his personality, his life and his appearance:

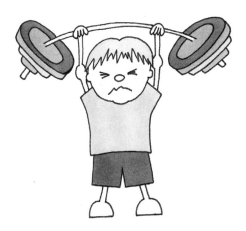

Where do you think we get this idea about how guys 'should' be? How realistic is this?

How many people do you think actually look and act like this picture?

Do you think you should look and act like this? How does that make you feel?

Thinking about Body Image

What messages do you hear from your **mother** (or closest adult female) about her body image or your body? For example, is she always talking about going on a diet, or does she think you shouldn't wear what you want to wear?

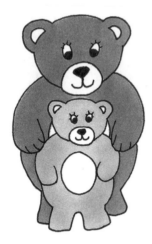

What messages do your **friends** give you about body image? For example, are they always saying they look fat or criticising other girls' appearances? How does that make you feel about your body?

Challenging Negative Body-related Thoughts

List below some of the negative things you say to yourself that can erode your self-esteem.

Self-critical thoughts What you say to yourself.	Consequences How does that thought make you feel about yourself? How does it make you behave?	Alternative thought Think of a more helpful and realistic thought that could replace the critical one.

Dispelling Diet Myths

Skipping meals does not help weight loss and dieting

Skipping meals or 'fasting' often leads to unhealthy eating patterns because you become so hungry that when you next allow yourself to eat you are likely to consume far more calories than if you had just eaten the missed meal in the first place.

When you skip a meal or two, your body, which has adapted to certain eating patterns, sends out the signal for fuel. No matter how good your will power is, you will give in eventually, and the foods you will choose are likely to be high in calories and of a large quantity.

High-protein diets are potentially dangerous

These popular diets focus on eating meat, fish, poultry and eggs while restricting carbo-hydrates (cereals, sugars). They can be dangerous because they can strain the kidneys and the liver. These diets can also be high in fat, which can be harmful. Restricting car-bohydrates can cause weakness, dizziness, nausea and dehydration. These types of diets can often deprive you of fibre, essential vitamins and minerals.

Low-calorie diets will actually make you put on weight

Diets that are made up of low-calorie foods (e.g. diet shakes) or consist of one food type that is very low in calories (e.g. grapefruit) are very harmful. While initially people might lose weight, this is usually fluid, and they will rapidly regain it, and more, when they begin eating normally.

Diet pills, cellulite creams and other gimmicks do NOT work

Medications designed to speed up your metabolism or suppress your appetite are DANGEROUS. Nothing will burn your fat away, rid you of cellulite or make your skin firmer and more toned, etc. Sweating in a sauna, wearing body wraps or rubber belts does NOTHING!!!

The final word on weight maintenance

The only things that will make your body fit and healthy are a **balanced diet** and **moderate, safe exercise**. There are no quick fixes or easy answers. Just look after your body, treat it with respect, and maintain its health responsibly.

8.3 Staying on track

This section focuses on staying on track, being aware of possible problems that could occur in the future, and how to deal with them. The exercises encourage young clients and their families to use positive thinking, to utilise the support of others when needed, and how to be aware of signs that they may need more help to prevent possible relapse.

Power Thoughts

Suitable for: any age

For children and adolescents, positive, 'brave' thoughts could be put onto the cards on this sheet (especially if it has been photocopied onto coloured card and decorated!). They can then put these cards in their pocket and carry them with them throughout the day. This way, child and adolescent clients can read their positive thoughts any time they need to. If the child decorates their cards and names them, they are more likely to refer to them in times of need.

Making Good Decisions

Suitable for: older children and adolescents

This sheet outlines how to make good decisions for young people. It complements the problem-solving sheet ('What to Do?' on page 81 in Section 2.6, Problem-solving) and guides them through the steps of defining the problem, listing possible solutions, looking at the advantages and disadvantages of each option, and selecting and planning the best option. This may provide a visual prompt for the therapist to use when helping children to make difficult decisions.

The Future Me

Suitable for: older children and adolescents

This sheet asks children and adolescents to think about the kind of person they would like to be when they are older (25 years old). It encourages them to think about the personal qualities they would like to possess as well as the strengths, talents and skills they would like to acquire. This can lead to valuable discussion about dreams and goals and the decisions they might need to make in order to achieve those goals.

What Keeps you Bouncing Back?

Suitable for: any age

This sheet simply asks clients to think about the things that keep them positive and happy in life. Brainstorming in this way might help the young client to see the positive influences in their life; so that they can better utilise them when they need to.

People to Lean on

Suitable for: any age

This sheet asks clients to think about the people they can go to when they need support or help. This sheet could be stuck on the wall in their bedroom or put on display in another visible location so that they can be constantly reminded of the people who care about them and are there to support them. It might be useful for the therapist to talk with the child about how they can ask for help from each of the people on their sheet and what sorts of problems each person might be able to assist them with, so that they know who to go to for which particular need.

Warnings

Suitable for: older children and adolescents

This sheet asks the older child or adolescent client (or the parents of a younger child client) to identify signs that they may be slipping back into old patterns and might need to seek support from family, friends or even to return to therapy. The aim of this exercise is to increase the client's awareness of their behaviour and symptoms in order for them to act quickly and prevent relapse.

Power Thoughts

Power thoughts

_____
_____
_____
_____
_____
_____
_____
_____

Power thoughts

_____
_____
_____
_____
_____
_____
_____
_____

Power thoughts

_____
_____
_____
_____
_____
_____
_____

Power thoughts

_____
_____
_____
_____
_____
_____
_____

Making Good Decisions

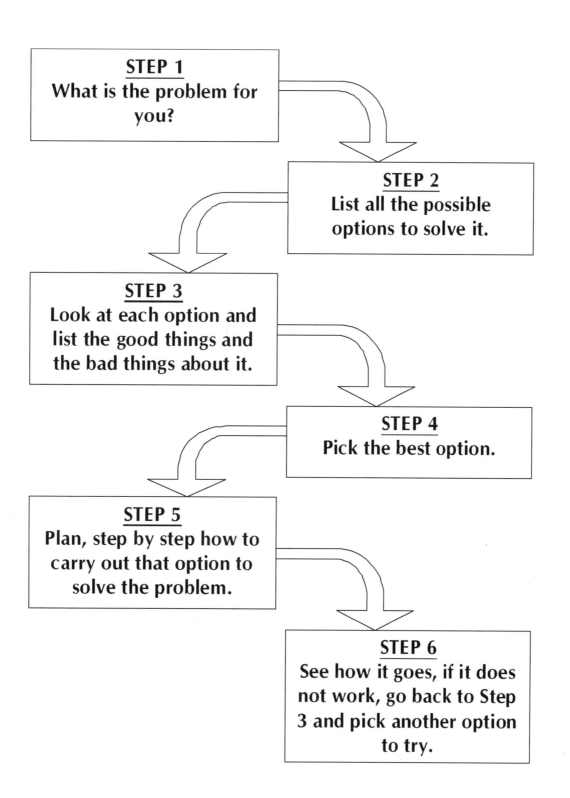

STEP 1
What is the problem for you?

STEP 2
List all the possible options to solve it.

STEP 3
Look at each option and list the good things and the bad things about it.

STEP 4
Pick the best option.

STEP 5
Plan, step by step how to carry out that option to solve the problem.

STEP 6
See how it goes, if it does not work, go back to Step 3 and pick another option to try.

The Future Me

What kind of person would you like to be in the future, say when you're 25 years old?

Describe on this sheet:

1.   What would you like to be doing with your life? _____

_____

_____

2.   What personal qualities would you like to have?

3.   What strengths/talents/skills would you like to have?

Personal qualities   Strengths/talents/skills

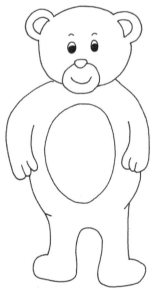

4.   What is your most important dream or goal for the future?

What Keeps You Bouncing Back?

What things help you to feel positive and motivated to achieve your goals?

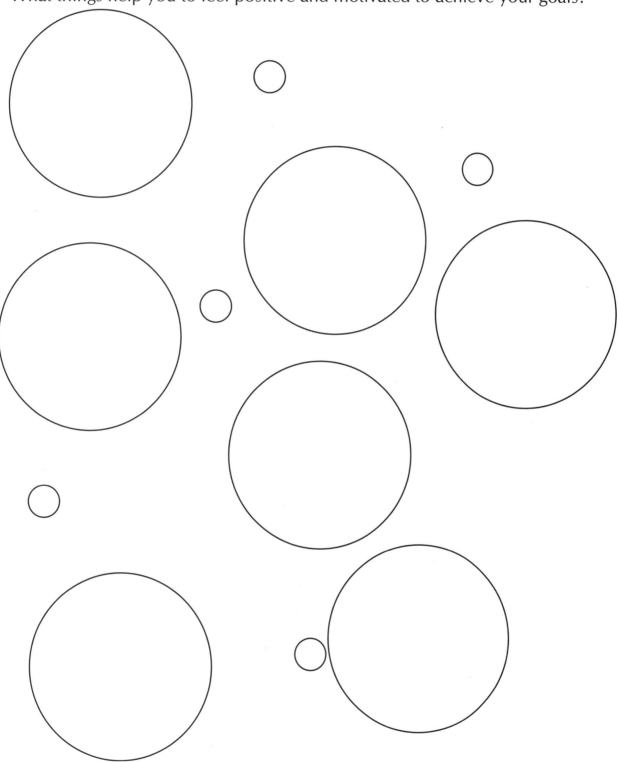

People to Lean on

Who can you go to for help when you need it? Write their names in the balloons!

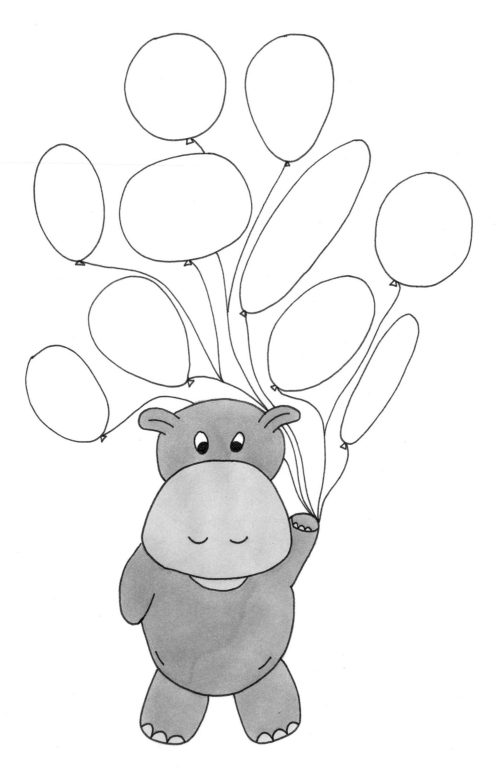

Warnings

How will you know when you might be slipping back into old patterns?

What signs will you notice in your body, thoughts and behaviour?

Will others be able to tell? How?

What do you need to do if you notice any of these warning signs?

Who can you go to for support if you need it?

Cool Connections with Cognitive Behavioural Therapy

Encouraging Self-esteem, Resilience and Well-being in Children and Young People Using CBT Approaches

Laurie Seiler

Paperback, ISBN 978 1 84310 618 0, 208 pages

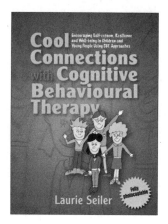

Cool Connections is an engaging programme that provides a cognitive behavioural therapy (CBT) approach to positively modifying the everyday thoughts, feelings and behaviours of children and young people aged 9 to 14, particularly those who are vulnerable or at risk.

Intended as an early intervention for use with children before they develop social, emotional or mental health difficulties, this programme combines a summary of CBT principles and step-by-step instructions with 10 sessions of games, handouts, home activities and therapeutic exercises designed to encourage resilience and self-esteem and reduce feelings of anxiety and depression.

Fully photocopiable, fully illustrated, flexible and easy to use, *Cool Connections with Cognitive Behavioural Therapy* is an effective tool for professionals working to improve the general well-being of children and young people, including psychologists, psychiatrists, counsellors, social workers, child and adolescent mental health services, and professionals in residential care settings and schools.

Listening to Children

A Practitioner's Guide

Alison McLeod

Paperback, ISBN 978 1 84310 549 7, 224 pages

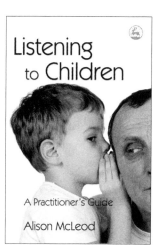

'Listening to children' is often understood differently by adults and the children they are supposed to be listening to: it involves not just paying attention to what young people say, but taking what they say seriously and acting in response.

Providing an introduction to the ideas behind listening to children and young people and how to do it, this guide offers a range of techniques for effective listening, encompassing observation and communication, explaining difficult issues, helping young people to talk about their experiences and involving them in decision-making. Good practice checklists, reflective exercises and quotations from children are given throughout, as well as a range of interdisciplinary practice examples showing situations where effective communication has been established with children.

Listening to Children is essential reading for professionals working with children and young people, and will be particularly useful for students in the fields of social care, health and education.

Anger Management Games for Children

Deborah M. Plummer

Illustrations by Jane Serrurier

Paperback, ISBN 978 1 84310 628 9, 160 pages

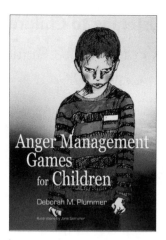

This practical handbook helps adults to understand, manage and reflect constructively on children's anger. Featuring a wealth of familiar and easy-to-learn games, it is designed to foster successful anger management strategies for children aged 5–12.

The book covers the theory behind the games in accessible language, and includes a broad range of enjoyable activities: active and passive, verbal and non-verbal, and for different sized groups. The games address issues that might arise in age-specific situations such as sharing a toy or facing peer pressure. They also encourage children to approach their emotions as a way to facilitate personal growth and healthy relationships.

This is an ideal resource for teachers, parents, carers and all those working with anger management in children.

Grief in Children

A Handbook for Adults
Second Edition

Atle Dyregrov
Foreword by Professor William Yule

Paperback, ISBN 978 1 84310 612 8, 208 pages

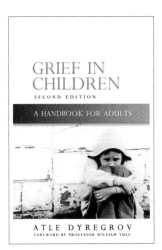

This fully updated second edition of *Grief in Children* explains children's understanding of death at different ages and provides information on how the adults around them can best help them cope.

Whether a child experiences the death or loss of a friend, family member, classmate or teacher, it is important for those caring for a bereaved child to know how to respond to their needs. Illustrated with vignettes, this accessible guide explores the methods of approaching grief that have been shown to work, provides advice on how loss and bereavement should be handled at school, explains when it is appropriate to enlist expert professional help and discusses the value of support for children and caregivers.

Speaking about the Unspeakable

Non-Verbal Methods and Experiences
in Therapy with Children

Edited by Dennis McCarthy
Foreword by Priscilla Rodgers

Paperback, ISBN 978 1 84310 879 5, 160 pages

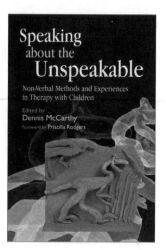

Children do not always have the capacity or need to express themselves through words. They often succeed in saying more about their feelings and experiences by communicating non-verbally through play and other expressive, creative activities.

The basic premise of *Speaking about the Unspeakable* is that life's most pivotal experiences, both good and bad, can be truly expressed via the language of the imagination. Through creativity and play, children are free to articulate their emotions in a more effective way. The contributors, all experienced child therapists, describe a wide variety of non-verbal therapeutic techniques, including clay, sand, movement and nature therapy, illustrating their descriptions with moving case studies from their professional experience.

Accessible and engaging, this book will inspire child psychologists and therapists, art therapists and anyone with an interest in therapeutic work with children.